WRITING SKILLS FOR VETERINARIANS

WRITING SKILLS FOR VETERINARIANS

Ryane E. Englar, DVM, DABVP (Canine and Feline Practice)

Assistant Professor and Clinical Education Coordinator
Kansas State University College of Veterinary Medicine
Manhattan, KS

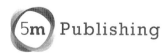 Publishing

Published by
5M Publishing Ltd,
Benchmark House,
8 Smithy Wood Drive,
Sheffield, S35 1QN, UK
Tel: +44 (0) 1234 81 81 80
www.5mpublishing.com

A Catalogue record for this book is available from the British Library

ISBN 9781789180350

Book layout by
Keystroke, Neville Lodge, Tettenhall, Wolverhampton

Printed by Replika Press Pvt Ltd, India

Photos by the author unless otherwise indicated

Contents

About the Author

Ryane E. Englar, DVM, DABVP (Canine and Feline Practice) graduated from Cornell University College of Veterinary Medicine in 2008. She practiced as an associated veterinarian in a companion animal clinic for five years before transitioning into the educational realm as an advocate for pre-clinical training in primary care. She began her debut in academia as a Clinical Instructor of the Community Practice Service at Cornell University's Hospital for Animals. She then transitioned into the role of Assistant Professor as founding faculty at Midwestern University College of Veterinary Medicine. Midwestern University granted her the opportunity to pave the way for the inaugural Class of 2018 by building something out of nothing – a beacon of opportunity within the desolate desert of Arizona. She joined the faculty at Kansas State University in May 2017 to design and debut a Clinical Skills curriculum. Her research areas of interest include clinical communication and educational outcomes. When she is not facilitating student learning or advancing primary care, she trains in the art of ballroom dancing and competes nationally with her instructor, Lowell E. Fox.

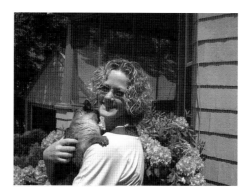

Preface

As veterinary educators, we are tasked with the impossible: to instill in our students all the skills that they require to be successful in clinical practice.

This is a tall order.

As someone who graduated proudly from Cornell University College of Veterinary Medicine in 2008, I can attest to the fact that I was delivered into private practice with "book smarts," but not "street smarts." That is, I had the knowledge base to excel. What I lacked was the follow-through.

I had not quite developed mastery over how to translate my knowledge into tangible skills surrounding patient care.

I was no different from any other new graduate. On graduation day, we were all works in progress at various stages of refinement.

The truth is that no one institution can cover it all. No one educator can teach it all.

Learning any trade takes time. The teacher in me believes that learning veterinary medicine takes time and a half.

As a practicing veterinarian, I held patients' lives in my hands. That action came with a certain degree of responsibility and the commitment to improve.

I worked hard to remedy my deficiencies so as not to compromise patient care. The truth is that all of us in veterinary medicine work hard.

We take the time to develop our surgical skills so that we operate with great finesse.

We devote time to continuing education to improve our mastery of specialty medicine.

But we rarely devote the time, both in our veterinary education and beyond, to the basics.

We rarely consider that which is most essential to patient care. For instance, we rarely pursue, in depth, how to perform a comprehensive physical examination. With even less frequency, we address the need for improvements in medical documentation.

In most veterinary schools, medical documentation is a lost art. It is an afterthought. It is something that we assume students will pick up on in their clinical year.

Unfortunately, what most of us pick up on are bad habits, if anything.

At the end of the day, we still see patient records as an obstacle: something that keeps us in the clinic after hours, something that we have to get through in order to get home.

Yet written communication is an essential component of patient care. It is a determinant of patient outcomes because it serves as a record of what happened to the patient and when. In this respect, written communication is the key to case management and continuity of care.

Written communication makes sure that everyone who is involved in patient care is on the same page.

Written communication bonds us as clinicians to our clients in a promise of partnership. It is a record of our contract to one another in terms of what we have agreed upon and why.

Written communication tracks patient progress. It also holds us legally responsible for our actions when patient progress goes awry. There is a saying in medicine: "If it isn't written, it didn't happen."

Written communication sets a standard for the practice of veterinary medicine. As educators we need to do a better job of emphasizing this standard and supporting student growth in this arena in the same way as we would encourage surgical training.

To produce Day-One ready graduates, we need to return to the basics.

No matter how much the profession evolves in terms of knowledge and technology, we are only as good as the imprint that we leave behind in the form of the patient record.

Medical documentation may not be the most entertaining of topics, but I challenge you to see it in a different light.

Just as a complete blood count (CBC) can be diagnostic, I encourage you to think of the medical record as both a resource and a tool that helps you to find patient-specific answers.

Dedication

Instructional coach Sean Junkins once said that:

> So often you find that the students you're trying to inspire are the ones that end up inspiring you.

In February 2014, I was invited to join a small core of founding faculty and build Midwestern University College of Veterinary Medicine in Glendale, Arizona, from the ground up.

If you have never had the opportunity to be in on the ground level of a giant feat, it is difficult to describe the level of energy and excitement that buzzed around campus in those days.

Imagine a chance of a lifetime: an opportunity to start with a clean slate, to build something from nothing, to be constrained by nothing but one's imagination.

When I arrived that February, ground had not yet been broken on the veterinary campus.

Students had been interviewed, offers of matriculation had been made, and the Class of 2018 had accepted their place in the history books as the first of its kind.

But I had yet to meet The Students.

For the first six months of my employment at Midwestern, there was only a group of us faculty.

We shared a dream that became our compass, our reason for being.

We dreamed the college into being.

We dreamed of the day when students would arrive on campus and fill the corridors.

We dreamed of the day when they would soak up our knowledge and rise from the ashes of the desert to become Great Veterinarians.

Like most educators, I had hoped that I would change their lives.

What I did not count on was just how much they had changed me.

In the years that followed, I came to know them all as my "Kids."

They became more than names on a class roster.

They were more than the faces that stared back at me.

Over the days, weeks, months, and years, they became a part of my heart.

To this day, they motivate me.

They taught me how to teach, and how to open up my heart to other people.

They taught me the power of faith in one other: they taught me to believe in myself the way that I believed in them.

To this day, they are my inspiration.

For that reason, this textbook belongs to them. They are who breathed it into being.

They are the reason that I will never regret my time at Midwestern University.

They are, and always will be, the reason that I consider Arizona *home*.

To my inaugural class, the Class of 2018 –
for breathing the dream of Midwestern into a breathtaking reality.

You represent Hope.

To my second-born, the Class of 2019 –
for furthering the dream into unforeseen directions.

You represent Growth.

To my third-born, the Class of 2020 –
for being light amidst the dark and a reminder that good prevails.

You represent New Beginnings.

Respectfully yours,
Dr. E
=^..^=

Acknowledgments

I have the best family in the whole world. Everybody says that, but how many of us truly believe it?

Each day, every day, I am thankful for my nuclear family: my mother, Jill; my father, Richard; and my brother, Brent.

This core of loved ones has watched me grow and transform over the years.

They loved me then as they love me now.

They also blessed me with the belief that, as life goes on, we choose to expand whom we consider family. They taught me to add to my collection, to fill up my heart with positive energy, to make our family a wider circle based upon trust.

Richard Bach once wrote that:

 The bond that links your true family is not one of blood,
 but of respect and joy in each other's life.

Because my nuclear family nurtured that philosophy, I have many *families.*

At this time, I would like to acknowledge my *dance family.*

Those who knew me prior to February 2014 would have never described me as a dancer. As a child, I practically kicked myself out of ballet.

I never thought that I would dream of a waltz in the middle of the night, or that I would listen to a new pop hit on the radio and think, what kind of dance would I dance to this?

I never thought that I would fall in love with ballroom.

I never thought I could be anything but a veterinarian, a doctor of science . . . someone who fixed cats and dogs and taught others how to practice medicine.

I love veterinary medicine. I will always love veterinary medicine. But I didn't know then what I know now: I didn't have to limit myself. I didn't have to choose.

For their role in changing my perspective, I would like to acknowledge my *dance family*, Arrowhead Arthur Murray, who entered my life in January 2014.

Arrowhead unlocked the door to a new and exciting world in which, much like veterinary medicine, learning was endless.

When Lowell E. Fox joined Arrowhead and became my permanent instructor in July

2014, he built me as a dancer from the ground up. He accepted me for who I was and, in an uncanny sort of way, knew who I would become.

Under Arrowhead's wings, I did grow. I learned my steps. I learned to feel the music, and I learned to trust. I learned to close my eyes and listen to the movement of my dance partner rather than words, and I learned that it was okay to fall as long as you got back up.

But you see the beauty is that Arrowhead didn't just teach me about dance, it taught me about life.

Thank you, Team Arrowhead, and thank you to Lowell, for teaching me what it means to live fully, freely, and boldly, without regret.

From Our First Choreographed Dance Routine (October 2014) . . .

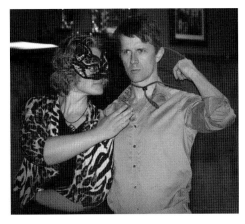

Courtesy of Steven Stringham Photography

. . . To Our Pro-Am Partnership in Ballroom Competitions (July 2017)

Thank you, Lowell, for the memories that will last a lifetime.

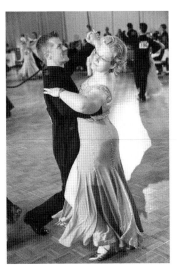

Courtesy of Maude Productions

Chapter 1

Introduction to Medical Documentation

We rely on documentation in everyday life. Purchases, large or small, are documented by receipts. International travel requires proper documentation to gain entry to other countries, and legal documentation is necessary to officiate a wedding, execute a living will, or grant power of attorney. Just as documents are a way for us to navigate personal circumstances, they also serve as a means by which colleagues communicate within a profession.

How a profession speaks through writing varies depending upon the discipline. For example, those who author English language or comparative literature manuscripts follow the Modern Language Association (MLA) style.(1) Likewise, medical disciplines adhere to their own set of rules when documenting provider–provider or provider–patient dialogue.(2–5) The profession of veterinary medicine shares this common need to communicate what constitutes patient care and how care for any given patient evolves.(6)

Learning how to communicate in writing as a clinician takes practice and attention to detail. Medical documentation may be tedious, yet it is no different than any other skill: it is capable of being learned and refined.(7)

As a veterinary student, I disconnected myself from viewing the medical record as a skill. To me, clinical skills were tangibly linked to patient outcomes: clinical skills were synonymous with clinical procedures – they were about doing something actively rather than passively writing. I dreamed of the day when I would perform surgery or dentistry. I never once dreamed of the day when I would make an entry into a veterinary medical record. However, medical documentation is just as important as drawing blood or taking a radiograph. It may not be exciting in the moment, but proper documentation is the vehicle by which we as clinicians guarantee that quality care was offered, accepted, and received.(8)

1.1 The "So What?" Factor: Why Medical Documentation Matters

If students view medical documentation as just another academic exercise, then it will always be an afterthought. Educators may unconsciously perpetuate this message by teaching it "on the fly" during clinical rotations, where patient care and record-keeping overlap. However, if educators can present medical documentation as an essential clinical tool that stimulates critical thinking, then students are more likely to recognize its value. Understanding how effective medical documentation contributes to case management is an important first step towards strengthening the profession's commitment to being thorough and complete.

In veterinary medicine, documentation matters most to the following entities:

- The patient
- The client
- The veterinarian

- The veterinary team
- The scientific community
- The law.

From both the *patient* and *client* perspective, documentation matters because it is a written record of the care that was received.(8) It can also be referenced when considering how patient care should proceed. For example, after a hospitalized patient is discharged from the clinic, the client may telephone to clarify when the next dose of medication "x" is due. This question is easily addressed by referring back to the patient's medical record. Complete documentation will include medication "x," its dose, dosing frequency, dosing route, and the time that it was last administered. In this case, documentation promotes compliance and minimizes the risk of accidental under- or overdosing.

From the *veterinarian's* perspective, documentation matters because it is a way to work through each clinical case, justify decision-making, record diagnostic and therapeutic interventions, and make adjustments to care based upon patient response to treatment.(9) For example, suppose a patient is admitted to the hospital for observation following a one-time episode of vomiting. The clinician will mull over the history and physical examination findings to determine which diagnoses are most likely and will advise the client accordingly. The clinician will keep track of certain vital parameters based upon an index of suspicion and will document trends. As the patient's clinical presentation evolves, so, too, does the clinician's plan of attack. What was once considered as a differential diagnosis may be ruled in or ruled out depending upon the patient's progress or diagnostic test results. Documentation thereby serves a purpose: a way to foster critical thinking about case patterns and decision-making.

Documentation is also a way for veterinarians to protect against faulty memory – theirs or the client's. Consider a recently adopted, indoor/outdoor, 12-week-old, female spayed, domestic shorthaired kitten that is new to the practice. History reveals that the kitten is acclimating into a multi-cat household, eating and drinking well, and using the litter box without issue. However, physical examination reveals epiphora and an isolated sneeze.

The veterinarian alerts the client that upper respiratory infections are common in kittens and that the stress of transitioning to a new household is often an inciting factor. The client is told to watch for a runny nose, lethargy, and inappetence because these could be signs that an infection has taken hold. In addition, the veterinarian reviews proper nutrition, vaccination protocols, and serological status with the client, and makes recommendations for topical flea preventative, fecal analysis, and microchipping. The client agrees to drop off a stool sample, but fails to follow through.

Three weeks later, the client contacts the clinic because spaghetti-like worms are in the litter box and she is frustrated: "No one told me that my Ginger could have worms!"

If I were the clinician in this case, I would not recall with certainty what transpired three weeks ago. I would assume that gastrointestinal parasites were discussed, but there is no place for assumptions when it comes to patient care or customer service in the healthcare industry.

In this case, documentation provides instant recall. A cursory review of the medical record outlines that yes, in fact, the possibility of gastrointestinal parasites was discussed with the client and that yes, in fact, she was encouraged to hand-deliver a stool sample and administer prophylactic dewormer.

The clinician could then follow up to clarify if dewormer was administered or, if not, why? Is there a patient compliance issue? If so, it is important to establish this early on so that strategies for administering medication can be discussed before additional doses are missed. In this way, documentation serves as a record of client education: what was discussed with the client and what the client did or did not agree to.(7)

From the perspective of the *veterinary team*, documentation provides for continuity of care within a practice. For example, colleagues frequently inherit other clinicians' cases when they call out sick, are attending a conference, or are away on vacation. These cases do not run themselves in the absence of the original attending clinician. Transferring patient care to a clinician who has access to a complete medical record is advantageous. Record review should uncover the rationale for ongoing treatments as well as outline which parameters are being assessed to evaluate patient status. By reviewing the record and tracking the patient care plan, diagnostic tests are not unnecessarily repeated and the client is kept in the loop regarding diagnostic test results.

Documentation also assists with recheck appointments that, for various reasons, are not scheduled with the veterinarian that made the initial diagnosis. Consider the colleague who has inherited a recheck appointment for chronic dermatitis. This veterinarian may have little to no relationship with the patient or client, and little to no firsthand knowledge of what transpired at the initial consultation. A complete medical record provides key insight into how the patient presented, in order for the veterinarian to make educated decisions about whether the patient has improved or regressed.(10)

It is equally important to maintain continuity of care between practices. Second-opinion cases and referrals to board-certified veterinary specialists are common. Both scenarios require facilities to communicate with one another via medical records to demonstrate the flow of care, what has and has not been done to address the presenting complaint, and where to go from here.

If a patient from Practice "A" presents to Practice "B" for a second opinion for chronic diarrhea, documentation from Practice "A" provides Practice "B" with a starting point. The veterinarian at Practice "B" will appreciate that the patient has already submitted to a complete blood count, a serum chemistry panel, a fecal float, and one round of metronidazole therapy that started on day "w," at dose "x," at "y" dosing frequency, for "z" number of days.

The secondary provider should receive the results of each test as well as an outline of the patient's response to treatment. This transparency on paper prevents unnecessary duplication of effort and facilitates decision-making about next steps. Skillful management of cases and consumer satisfaction often stem from the perception of organization and easy-to-retrieve data.(10)

From the perspective of the *scientific community*, documentation matters because it provides data that fuels the research industry and paves the way for an evidence-based approach to clinical medicine.(10, 11) Consider, for example, *Borrelia burgdorferi*, the causative agent of Lyme disease. Veterinary medical records and national databases provide information about this emerging disease, its prevalence, and its geographical distribution.(12–14) Much of what is known today about Lyme disease can be traced back to case studies that link the development of antibodies to *B. burgdorferi* to clinical disease.(15–26) Without documentation to record the clinical presentation and diagnostic work-up, Lyme disease may not have been linked to arthropathy or nephropathy.(15, 19, 21, 23) Without documentation of host responses to *B. burgdorferi* and without documentation to trace the serological prevalence of the causative agent over time, there may not have been a push for the development of a Lyme vaccination. Vaccinations arise from a need, and evidence to support that need resides in the medical record.

From the perspective of the *law*, documentation matters because it is a legal record of patient care: what happened, what did not, and why.(8, 11) The medical record exists to protect the patient from substandard care. When the quality of patient care and/or the competence of the attending clinician is called into question, it is the completeness of the medical record that dictates whether the standard of care was met.(8)

Standard of care is not static: it evolves over time as the profession's knowledge grows. Local, regional, national, and international organizations set guidelines for clinical practice that are in tune with legislation. These guidelines vary from country to country and between continents depending upon legislation, species serviced, and the context of a given clinical scenario. As evidence-based medicine paves the way for scientific discoveries and improved understanding – for example, the need to provide analgesia in addition to anesthesia – guidelines change shape and form. In this way, they are malleable. They may shift based upon changes in cultural and ethical perspectives.

Global organizations that weigh in on veterinary standard of care include, but are not limited to, the:

- Association of Shelter Veterinarians (ASV)
- International Association for Aquatic Animal Medicine (IAAAM)
- International Veterinary Academy of Pain Management (IVAPM)
- World Organisation for Animal Health (OIE)
- World Small Animal Veterinary Association (WSAVA)
- World Veterinary Association (WVA).

Within the United Kingdom (U.K.), both the British Veterinary Association (BVA) and the British Small Animal Veterinary Association (BSAVA) play important roles in setting high standards for clinical practice.

The Animal Welfare Foundation (AWF) was founded by members of the BVA. Both groups work together to address ethical issues, particularly those involving production animal medicine, such as the transport of livestock and animal welfare at time of slaughter.

The Canadian Veterinary Medical Association (CVMA) also helps to define standards within the profession. The CVMA serves as the voice of the Canadian veterinary team. In addition to the CVMA, Canadian veterinarians rely upon regional governing bodies within their individual provinces, such as the Ontario Veterinary Medical Association (OVMA) and the College of Veterinarians of Ontario (CVO).

In the United States (U.S.), key players include, but are not limited to, the:

- American Animal Hospital Association (AAHA)
- American Association of Bovine Practitioners (AABP)
- American Association of Equine Practitioners (AAEP)
- American Association of Feline Practitioners (AAFP)
- American Association of Swine Veterinarians (AASV)
- American Board of Veterinary Practitioners (ABVP)
- American Veterinary Medical Association (AVMA)
- AVMA American Board of Veterinary Specialties (ABVS).

Within the U.S., state governing boards and state veterinary practice acts provide additional guidelines concerning practice standards.(27)

All aforementioned organizations value patient safety and the patient–provider relationship. Documentation is a way to protect both. Effective documentation is protective against liability whereas ineffective documentation invites it.(8)

Documentation is not an exercise in futility. It definitively impacts patient care, patient outcomes, and client satisfaction. It also affects our interactions with other members of the veterinary community, and how they perceive us.

In order that documentation's impact be positive, it must be complete and accurate. What actions clinicians take to provide and manage patient care must match what is in the medical record.(28)

There is a paucity of research in the veterinary medical literature that evaluates this aspect of clinical practice. However, recent studies in human medicine suggest that neither medical students nor physicians exhibit best practice when it comes to documentation.(28–34)

Under-documentation is more common than over-documentation, with a tendency to omit key physical exam findings.(29, 31) A study by Dresselhaus et al. cited an under-documentation rate of 20.5% for human medical physicians following standardized patient encounters.(35, 36)

Medical students are not immune to errors of omission. A 2009 study by Szauter et al. compared 207 student-led standardized patient encounters to their associated medical records. Records were incomplete and/or inaccurate in 96% of cases.(28)

It is likely that the veterinary profession experiences similar deficiencies in documentation. This may be due to limited internal regulation. Short of veterinary licensing board complaints and litigation, there is very little motivation in everyday practice to audit records on a regular basis, if at all. Unlike the review process that basic scientists and researchers endure when presenting a manuscript for publication, veterinary medical records are not routinely analyzed for errors. They do not routinely undergo peer review. Practitioners may gripe about others' work, particularly when deciphering it makes more work for themselves. However, there is rarely, if ever, formalized review beyond clinical rotations in veterinary school.

Veterinarians are required to engage in continuing education (CE) to improve and/or clarify their knowledge base. Given that medical documentation is a technical skill, it, too, could benefit from refresher courses or other programs affiliated with CE. Self-directed and/or group-inspired learning have the potential to be invaluable. They may curb bad habits before they become fatal flaws in front of the licensing board.(10) They could also help to correct questionable practices before they compromise patient care or provider reputation.

1.2 Which Key Attributes Strengthen Medical Documentation?

In order for medical documentation to be effective, it should be: (7, 9, 11)

- Credible
- Clear
- Concise.

Clinicians demonstrate *credibility* through the sharing of facts. Facts should be stated as objectively as possible without straying into the subjective, making assumptions, reading between the lines, or implying something untoward. Facts should not be embellished: they are what they are and leave no room for fiction.(9, 11) Consider a situation in which a veterinarian fails to ask the client if the patient has had adverse reactions to antibiotics in the past. The veterinarian should document that the issue of adverse events was not discussed rather than writing "no known drug allergies" in the medical record. The latter implies that the veterinarian asked, and received an answer when in fact that conversation never occurred.(31)

Clinicians demonstrate *clarity* by using medical terms and abbreviations correctly, and by eliminating vague language. The meaning of any word, phrase, or sentence should be immediately clear to the reader without the need for clarification.(9, 11) For example, a new client may ask about the appropriate age for a puppy to undergo elective ovariohysterectomy (OVH). This may invite discussion about the procedure itself, what it entails, and the recovery time, as well as anticipated risks versus benefits. Following the consultation, the veterinarian may be prone to document the following in the medical record: "Discussed OVH; owner elects to proceed."

Weeks from now, what does that statement mean? What was discussed and why? How likely is the clinician to remember?

Cloudy recall gives rise to faulty assumptions. The clinician may incorrectly assume that cost, anesthetic risk, overnight hospitalization, and aftercare were discussed. This discrepancy muddies the water when it comes to informed consent: sufficient information may not have been provided to allow the client to make an informed decision.(37)

Clarity of documentation requires careful word choice. "Watch for pain" may be intuitive for the clinician who writes it in the discharge summary; however, have the signs of pain been spelled out for the client, who will be observing the patient at home? An improvement would be to replace "watch for" with "re-examine if," followed by a list of clinical signs that the client is capable of identifying.

"Re-examine if" is a helpful phrase that guides patient care. For example, a dog may have presented to the veterinary clinic for acute onset of emesis. After an unremarkable physical examination, the client may have elected to hold off on diagnostic testing and take the dog home for observation. But what exactly is the client watching for?

"Re-examine if" provides clarity. For example, "re-examine if" the dog:

- Vomits blood
- Vomits within 60 minutes of eating or drinking
- Vomits more than twice overnight
- Refuses the next three meals.

Spelling contributes to clarity as well.(9, 11) Colleagues may understand what is meant by pruritis [*sic*]. In fact, pruritus is misspelled as pruritis [*sic*] in 5% of articles indexed in PubMed.(38) However, some distinctions are not readily apparent, particularly when phrases are taken out of context. Ileum and ilium, for example, refer to two very different anatomical structures. The former refers to the distal portion of small bowel, as compared to the latter, a skeletal component of the bony pelvis. In the context of a phrase or sentence, the reader can infer which structure is being discussed. Out of context, the meaning becomes appreciably less clear.

In some clinical scenarios, clarity requires specific details. The body, for instance, does not just have one bladder. There is the urinary bladder and the gall bladder. Out of context, writing "the bladder was palpable" does little to clarify the clinician's meaning. The clinician most likely means that the *urinary* bladder was palpable, which is normally felt on physical examination, as compared to the *gall* bladder, which is not. However, relying upon assumptions can lead to dangerous mistakes. The patient with a palpable *gall* bladder requires immediate medical, if not surgical, attention. In this case, clarity would be improved by writing, "the urinary bladder was palpably normal."

Clarity is also achieved by avoiding sudden shifts in tense.(9) Consider, for example, the following series of statements: "Was unable to stand on own. Is weight-bearing lame. Circled to the right. Walks with hesitation."

This documentation may confuse the reader because the timeline is unclear. Do the first and third statements refer to the patient's presentation at home? Do the second and fourth statements describe the patient's presentation at the clinic? When was the patient unable to stand? Is the patient still circling now? Which actions happened in the past and which are still occurring? Without more information to fill in the blanks, these descriptions are less than helpful and the reader is required to interpret what is written. Different interpretations may lead the case down very different paths.

Note that the need for clarity in documentation also depends upon the audience. For whom is the written material intended?

Discharge summaries that go home to the client with the patient need to be exceptionally clear. This ensures a smooth transition in continuity of care from the clinic to home environment. Because clients are less likely to understand medical jargon, clarity is essential. When writing discharge statements, consider trading out medical terminology for appropriate colloquial terms, write:

- "blue gums" instead of cyanosis
- "neuter" instead of castration
- "nose bleed" instead of epistaxis
- "spay" instead of ovariohysterectomy
- "straining to urinate" instead of stranguria
- "trouble breathing" instead of dyspnea
- "vomiting" instead of emesis.

Save medical jargon for correspondence between members of the veterinary team. If referring the patient to a specialist, it is appropriate to reference appropriate medical terminology on the referral form so that you both can be on the same page. For example:

- "Anisocoria, with aqueous flare"
- "Negative PLR OS; sluggish PLR OD"
- "Progressive left-sided paraparesis"
- "Stress hyperglycemia with glucosuria"
- "Stuporous mentation"
- "Syncopal episodes after exertion"
- "Three-month history of polyuria/polydipsia."

Clinicians demonstrate ***brevity*** by extracting key ideas from the client-provided history and highlighting these in the medical record.(7) Consider the following excerpt from a canine patient's chart:

> Normal two days ago. Woke up yesterday and came over to the bowl in the kitchen for breakfast. Took a lick or two of canned food and then went back to bed. When food was brought over to him, he turned his head away. Refused all treats throughout the day, did not drink water, and did not show interest in eating dinner.

Although documentation is complete and paints a picture of the health status of the patient, it includes extraneous information that adds unnecessary bulk. The reader must work hard to extract what is important from the rest of the words on the page.

A more concise approach to the case might be to document that the patient was:

OK until yesterday. Interested in breakfast, but did not eat. Subsequently food-averse. Refused treats, water, and dinner. Lethargic.

The key facts of the case have been captured without the reader having to sift through extraneous information that is not vital to the outcome of the case.

Note the importance of being brief without being incomplete.

Before excluding information, ask yourself whether having access to it will alter your clinical acumen. For instance, when evaluating an anorexic patient, it is important to include a diet history, including any recent changes in diet, as well as whether the patient is vomiting. Failing to elicit this information from the client and failing to document the client's responses would abbreviate the medical record in a way that makes it incomplete.

Being credible, clear, and concise strengthen the quality of medical documentation. Quality record-keeping facilitates patient care and follow-up and decreases the potential for miscommunication between veterinary providers and their clients.

1.3 Which Errors Weaken Medical Documentation?

As occurs in every other type of writing, errors are bound to find their way into medical documentation. These may range from a benign typo to an inappropriate word choice or even an unintentional, but potentially devastating, piece of information, such as inaccurately transcribed laboratory data.

It is tempting to correct errors using methods that are approved in other disciplines. However, the use of correction fluid to "white out" errors and the use of scribbling over to "black out" errors is inappropriate in the medical field. The equivalent scenario for an electronic medical record would be hitting the delete key to erase any information that has been date- and time-stamped. Although these actions are typically well intentioned, they may appear as attempts to cover-up malpractice in the eyes of an outside observer or to a court of law.(9, 11, 27)

Rather than obliterate erroneous information, paper records can be annotated using a single or double strike-through with permanent ink, using a caret to insert words as needed, and initialing above the error with the date of correction. For larger corrections, a dated and initialed addendum can be made below the erroneous entry. The use of electronic medical records can also prevent record alteration by relying upon a computer system that limits access to and converts records into read-only files.(7, 9, 11, 27)

Just as removing data from files is inappropriate, it is equally improper to leave blank space.(9, 11) Blank space at the end of a line or between lines may be aesthetically pleasing; however, such spacing allows for the temptation to inappropriately introduce new material at a later date.

Consider how this might apply to a case of bilateral retinal detachment in a geriatric cat. The cat presents for acute onset of blindness. After the veterinarian confirms the cat's visual status, the distraught client files a complaint with the state licensing board. The client feels that no steps were taken by the veterinarian to identify the underlying disease state before it resulted in blindness. The cat had presented for a tech appointment once a month for the past three months for a nail trim and no one had ever noticed or mentioned the cat's declining vision to the client.

Fearing disciplinary action, the veterinarian reviews the medical record and sees that the cat's blood pressure was never taken or recorded at any of the visits that preceded the cat's blindness. If records are double-spaced, the veterinarian may be tempted to insert data after the fact, using a caret, to make it appear that standard of care was met.

To reduce this temptation, single-space records. In the event that handwritten documents contain unintentional blank spaces, draw a line or an "X" through them as deterrents against improper insertions.(9, 11)

Errors of omission also weaken medical documentation. Variations of the phrase, "if it isn't charted, it didn't happen,"(39) permeate the healthcare industry.(40–44)

As an example, let's reflect upon a case involving a recently adopted, yet fearful canine patient that presents for its initial wellness examination. On account of temperament, only a limited physical assessment can be performed. Rectal temperature, mucous membranes, and capillary refill time are not assessed. The clinician does not refer to them in the medical record or address why they are absent from it.

A month later, the dog presents to the emergency service in lateral recumbency with hemoabdomen. The patient is humanely euthanized and necropsy findings include a ruptured splenic mass. The distraught client files a complaint with the state licensing board because the primary clinician "missed" the diagnosis. The licensing board reviews the medical record, which is scant. There are no written explanations for the gaps in documentation.

Although the primary clinician recalls the case well and can explain why certain vital signs were not addressed at that initial visit, there is no evidence in writing that this is true. This is unfortunate for the clinician because outcomes of board complaints rest on proof rather than the veterinarian's recollection.(27)

Rather than risk disciplinary action, the veterinarian ought to think ahead. It is important to invest time documenting what did and did not occur, and why. The following statements are examples of transparency in explaining why certain variations of the *standard of care* physical examination was performed.

- "Rectal temperature was not taken because the cat presented in respiratory distress. Patient stabilization was prioritized and the cat was placed in an oxygen cage."
- "Oral exam was not performed because of temperament. A tongue depressor was used to lift the patient's lip folds through a basket muzzle to determine mucous membrane color, which was pink."

When in doubt, include it in the medical record.

Likewise, if something was missed, own up to it.

- "Blood pressure not taken at this visit due to time constraints. Contacted owner by telephone to request a follow-up visit within the next ____ weeks to obtain a value."

It is equally important to include recommendations that you made, even if the client does not wish to follow through.

- "Advised owner to pursue three-view thoracic radiographs as a 'met check.' Owner declined."
- "Recommended CBC/CHEM/UA as baseline labwork to evaluate organ health as part of the senior wellness check-up. Client cannot pursue today; will schedule in 2–3 months as able."

Firsthand data is essential, provided that it is accurate and conveyed without judgment. Firsthand data demonstrates what the member of the veterinary team encountered or witnessed. This paints a visual that can hold up in a court of law.

Secondhand data should not be inserted into the medical record unless it has been verified because so doing has the potential to propagate false information.(30) The "copy-and-paste" command has made this error commonplace in healthcare electronic medical records.(45) It is all too easy for the details from the last visit to be pasted to the present visit, and the details from today's visit to be pasted to a future visit. It becomes a chain reaction with the potential for adverse consequences.

Suppose, for instance, that a colleague incorrectly jots down laboratory findings as being "abnormal" at the last visit. If these lab values are not compared against the data and are assumed to be truth by the next clinician to pick up the patient file, then the patient may be erroneously labeled with a problem that does not exist. For example, miswriting the value for serum blood glucose may lead to an assumption that the patient is pre-diabetic. That assumption may lead to an unnecessary diagnostic work-up.

This scenario may seem far-fetched, but the copy-and-paste phenomenon is widespread in human healthcare. A 2008 anonymous survey questionnaire by Sharma et al. found that 40% of internists in the Northeastern United States copied laboratory values without double-checking, and 52% observed this behavior among colleagues.(30)

In addition, 22% have admitted to writing records for patients prior to an office visit or on a day when the office visit did not take place.(30) These errors of inclusion represent questionable documentation practices that threaten the credibility of the medical record and the integrity of the healthcare team.

END-OF-CHAPTER SUMMARY

Veterinary medical documentation benefits:

- The veterinary patient
- The veterinary client
- The veterinarian

- The veterinary team
- The scientific community
- The law.

Veterinary medical documentation should be:

- Clear
- Credible
- Concise.

Veterinary medical documentation is weakened by:

- Erasing data
- Omitting key data
- Inserting secondhand observations.

References

1. Mauk J, Metz J. The Composition of Everyday Life: A Guide to Writing. 5th ed. Australia; Boston, MA: Cengage Learning; 2016. xxxii, 781 pp.
2. Iverson C, American Medical Association. AMA Manual of Style: A Guide for Authors and Editors. 10th ed. Oxford; New York: Oxford University Press; 2007. xi, 1010 pp.
3. American Psychological Association. Publication Manual of the American Psychological Association. 6th ed. Washington, DC: American Psychological Association; 2010. xviii, 272 pp.
4. Buscher LS. Scientific Style and Format: the CSE Manual for Authors, Editors, and Publishers. 8th ed. Chicago, IL: University Of Chicago Press; 2014.
5. Taylor R. The Clinician's Guide to Medical Writing. New York, NY: Springer Science; 2005.
6. Christopher M, Young K. Writing for Publication in Veterinary Medicine: A Practical Guide for Researchers and Clinicians. John Wiley & Sons, Inc.; 2015. Available from: https//www.wiley.com/legacy/wileyblackwell/gmspdfs/VETWritingforPub/pubData/source/VETWritingforPubPDF.pdf
7. Borcherding S. Documentation Manual for Writing SOAP Notes in Occupational Therapy. 2nd ed. Thorofare, NJ: SLACK Incorporated; 2005.
8. Gutheil TG. Fundamentals of medical record documentation. Psychiatry (Edgmont). 2004;1(3):26–28.
9. Kettenbach G. Writing Patient/Client Notes: Ensuring Accuracy in Documentation. 4th ed. Philadelphia: F.A. Davis Company; 2004. 248 pp.

10. Weed LL. Medical records that guide and teach. 1968. MD Comput. 1993;10(2):100–114.

11. Rockett J, Lattanzio C, Christensen C. The Veterinary Technician's Guide to Writing SOAPS: A Workbook for Critical Thinking. Heyburn, Idaho: Rockett House Publishing LLC; 2013.

12. Bowman D, Little SE, Lorentzen L, Shields J, Sullivan MP, Carlin EP. Prevalence and geographic distribution of Dirofilaria immitis, Borrelia burgdorferi, Ehrlichia canis, and Anaplasma phagocytophilum in dogs in the United States: results of a national clinic-based serologic survey. Vet Parasitol. 2009;160(1–2):138–148.

13. Beichel E, Petney TN, Hassler D, Bruckner M, Maiwald M. Tick infestation patterns and prevalence of Borrelia burgdorferi in ticks collected at a veterinary clinic in Germany. Vet Parasitol. 1996;65(1–2):147–155.

14. Beall MJ, Chandrashekar R, Eberts MD, Cyr KE, Diniz PP, Mainville C, et al. Serological and molecular prevalence of Borrelia burgdorferi, Anaplasma phagocytophilum, and Ehrlichia species in dogs from Minnesota. Vector Borne Zoonotic Dis. 2008;8(4):455–464.

15. Levy SA, Magnarelli LA. Relationship between development of antibodies to Borrelia burgdorferi in dogs and the subsequent development of limb/joint borreliosis. J Am Vet Med Assoc. 1992;200(3):344–347.

16. Magnarelli LA, Anderson JF, Schreier AB, Ficke CM. Clinical and serologic studies of canine borreliosis. J Am Vet Med Assoc. 1987;191(9):1089–1094.

17. Levy SA, Duray PH. Complete heart block in a dog seropositive for Borrelia burgdorferi. Similarity to human Lyme carditis. J Vet Intern Med. 1988;2(3):138–144.

18. Magnarelli LA, Anderson JF, Kaufmann AF, Lieberman LL, Whitney GD. Borreliosis in dogs from southern Connecticut. J Am Vet Med Assoc. 1985;186(9):955–959.

19. Grauer GF, Burgess EC, Cooley AJ, Hagee JH. Renal lesions associated with Borrelia burgdorferi infection in a dog. J Am Vet Med Assoc. 1988;193(2):237–239.

20. Dambach DM, Smith CA, Lewis RM, Van Winkle TJ. Morphologic, immunohistochemical, and ultrastructural characterization of a distinctive renal lesion in dogs putatively associated with Borrelia burgdorferi infection: 49 cases (1987–1992). Vet Pathol. 1997;34(2):85–96.

21. Center SA, Smith CA, Wilkinson E, Erb HN, Lewis RM. Clinicopathologic, renal immunofluorescent, and light microscopic features of glomerulonephritis in the dog: 41 cases (1975–1985). J Am Vet Med Assoc. 1987;190(1):81–90.

22. Cohen ND, Carter CN, Thomas MA, Jr., Angulo AB, Eugster AK. Clinical and epizootiologic characteristics of dogs seropositive for Borrelia burgdorferi in Texas: 110 cases (1988). J Am Vet Med Assoc. 1990;197(7):893–898.

23. Koeman JP, Biewenga WJ, Gruys E. Proteinuria in the dog: a pathomorphological study of 51 proteinuric dogs. Res Vet Sci. 1987;43(3):367–378.

24. McKenna P, Clement J, Van Dijck D, Lauwerys M, Carey D, Van den Bogaard T, et al. Canine Lyme disease in Belgium. Veterinary Record. 1995;136(10):244–247.

25. Azuma Y, Kawamura K, Isogai H, Isogai E. Neurologic abnormalities in two dogs suspected Lyme disease. Microbiol Immunol. 1993;37(4):325–329.

26. Breitschwerdt EB, Nicholson WL, Kiehl AR, Steers C, Meuten DJ, Levine JF. Natural infections with Borrelia spirochetes in two dogs from Florida. J Clin Microbiol. 1994;32(2):352–357.

27. Wilson JF. Law and Ethics of the Veterinary Profession. Yardley, PA: Priority Press, Ltd.; 2000.

28. Szauter KM, Ainsworth MA, Holden MD, Mercado AC. Do students do what they write and write what they do? The match between the patient encounter and patient note. Acad Med. 2006;81(10 Suppl):S44–47.

29. Seo JH, Kong HH, Im SJ, Roh H, Kim DK, Bae HO, et al. A pilot study on the evaluation of medical student documentation: assessment of SOAP notes. Korean J Med Educ. 2016;28(2):237–241.

30. Sharma R, Kostis WJ, Wilson AC, Cosgrove NM, Hassett AL, Moreyra AE, et al. Questionable hospital chart documentation practices by physicians. J Gen Intern Med. 2008;23(11):1865–1870.

31. Worzala K, Rattner SL, Boulet JR, Majdan JF, Berg DD, Robeson M, et al. Evaluation of the congruence between students' postencounter notes and standardized patients' checklists in a clinical skills examination. Teach Learn Med. 2008;20(1):31–36.

32. Woodward CA, McConvey GA, Neufeld V, Norman GR, Walsh A. Measurement of physician performance by standardized patients. Refining techniques for undetected entry in physicians' offices. Med Care. 1985;23(8):1019–1027.

33. Luck J, Peabody JW, Dresselhaus TR, Lee M, Glassman P. How well does chart abstraction measure quality? A prospective comparison of standardized patients with the medical record. Am J Med. 2000;108(8):642–649.

34. Ellis PM, Blackshaw G, Purdie GL, Mellsop GW. Clinical information in psychiatric practice: what do doctors know, what do they think is known and what do they record? Med Educ. 1991;25(5):438–443.

35. Dresselhaus TR, Luck J, Peabody JW. The ethical problem of false positives: a prospective evaluation of physician reporting in the medical record. J Med Ethics. 2002;28(5):291–294.

36. Dresselhaus TR, Peabody JW, Lee M, Wang MM, Luck J. Measuring compliance with preventive care guidelines: standardized patients, clinical vignettes, and the medical record. J Gen Intern Med. 2000;15(11):782–788.

37. Owner Consent in Veterinary Medicine: American Veterinary Medical Association. Available from: https//www.avma.org/News/JAVMANews/Pages/070515e.aspx

38. Lehman JS. The problem with "pruritis". Arch Dermatol. 2010;146(2):203–204.

39. Trossman S. The documentation dilemma: Nurses poised to address paperwork burden. The American Nurse. 2001;33(5):1–18.

40. Page A, editor. Keeping Patients Safe: Transforming the Work Environment of Nurses. Institute of Medicine (US) Committee on the Work Environment for Nurses and Patient Safety. Washington, DC: National Academies Press; 2004. Available from: https://www.ncbi.nlm.nih.gov/pubmed/25009849

41. Nguyen AVT, Nguyen DA. Learning from Medical Errors: Legal Issues. Abingdon, United Kingdom: Radcliffe Publishing, Ltd.; 2005.

42. Andrews A, St Aubyn B. 'If it's not written down; it didn't happen.' Journal of Community Nursing. 2015;29(5):20–22.

43. Catalano J. Nursing Now! Today's Issues, Tomorrow's Trends. 7th ed. Philadelphia, PA: F.A. Davis Company; 2015.

44. David G, Vinkhuyzen E. Medical records' dynamic nature. If it isn't written down, it didn't happen. And if it is written down, it might not be what it seems. J AHIMA. 2013;84(11):32–35.

45. Hirschtick RE. A piece of my mind. Copy-and-paste. J Am Med Assoc. 2006;295(20):2335–2336.

Chapter 2

Learning the Lingo: The Language of Medical Documentation

Now that the mechanics of medical documentation have been reviewed, it is important to gain familiarity with the terminology that is commonly used. Medical terminology consists of descriptive words about the body, its physiology, pathology, and the procedures that can be performed.

Medical terminology can be tedious; however, it has a purpose. It exists to create a universal language in healthcare, one that is more precise and less likely to be misinterpreted. For example, a veterinarian may need to document a scar "below the hip." Without medical terminology to ground the discussion, that scar could be located virtually anywhere. "Below the hip" is a poor reference point. "Below the hip" could mean one centimeter below the hip or as far below the hip as the paw.

"Below the hip" also does not clarify other significant spatial relationships: is the scar along the front of the thigh, for instance, or is the scar behind the kneecap? Using medical terminology to define the location of the scar as being popliteal paints a very clear picture that the scar resides at the back of the knee. Medical terminology therefore contributes to clarity.

A comprehensive review of etymology is beyond the scope of this text and a basic working knowledge of medical jargon is assumed; however, recall that many medical terms stem from Greek or Latin languages. Recognizing the most commonly used roots, prefixes, and suffixes is an appropriate way for the novice to build a working vocabulary of medical jargon. Recall that the foundation of a word is a root. Prefixes attach onto the beginning of roots whereas suffixes attach onto the end of roots to alter the meaning of the word. For example, *myo* is the Greek prefix for muscle; *cardi* is the Greek root for heart; and *itis* is the Greek suffix for inflammation. All three words linked together form *myocarditis*, inflammation of the heart muscle.(1–6)

Refer to Tables 2.1–2.3 at the end of the chapter to review the most common medical prefixes, roots, and suffixes. Refer to medical and veterinary dictionaries and textbooks for more comprehensive lists.(1–6) It is important to consult these resources to clarify the meaning of words as needed to prevent misuse of medical terminology.

Medical terminology also includes descriptive words for directional terms and anatomical planes. Directional terms specify the location of one structure relative to another structure.(1, 3, 4) Think of the body of the patient as a map. Just as we would use the cardinal directions of north, south, east, and west to describe the location of one city relative to another, we use directional terms to point us in the right direction when describing body parts.

In order to make sense of directional terms, one must first recognize the anatomical names for parts of the body. For example, the veterinary equivalent of the human knee is the *stifle*. The human wrist is akin to the canine *carpus*, and the human ankle is the veterinary *tarsus*.(1, 3, 4)

Refer to Figures 2.1–2.3 to review the clinically relevant anatomy of the canine, equine, and bovine bodies. These figures are not intended to be comprehensive, but rather to provide an overview of the anatomy that is clinically relevant to medical documentation.

Note that body regions depicted in the canine photograph are named the same in the cat.

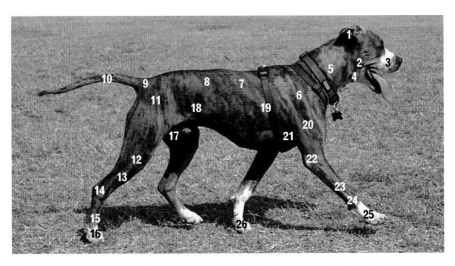

Figure 2.1 Canine external anatomy with labels. Courtesy of Analucia Aliaga

Key:

1. Ear	11. Upper thigh	21. Axilla (armpit)
2. Cheek	12. Stifle	22. Elbow
3. Muzzle	13. Crus	23. Antebrachium
4. Throat	14. Tarsus	24. Carpus
5. Neck	15. Metatarsus	25. Metacarpus
6. Shoulder	16. Hind paw	26. Forepaw
7. Back	17. Groin (inguinal region)	
8. Loin	18. Abdomen	
9. Tail set	19. Thorax	
10. Tail	20. Brachium	

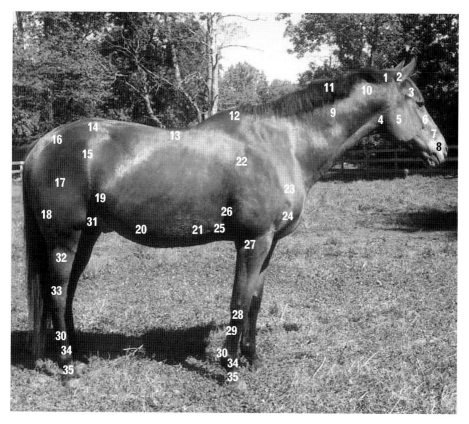

Figure 2.2 Equine external anatomy with labels. Courtesy of Sarah Ciamello

Key:

1. Poll	11. Mane	21. Barrel	31. Stifle
2. Ear	12. Withers	22. Shoulder	32. Gaskin
3. Forehead	13. Back	23. Point of shoulder	33. Hock
4. Throatlatch	14. Croup	24. Chest	34. Pastern
5. Cheek	15. Point of hip	25. Axilla	35. Hoof
6. Face	16. Buttock	26. Elbow	
7. Muzzle	17. Thigh	27. Forearm	
8. Nostril	18. Quarter	28. Knee	
9. Neck	19. Flank	29. Cannon	
10. Crest	20. Abdomen	30. Fetlock	

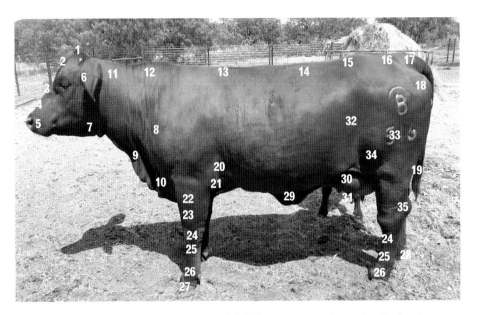

Figure 2.3 Bovine external anatomy with labels. Courtesy of Heather Bullard

Key:

1. Poll	11. Neck	21. Chest Floor	31. Teats
2. Forehead	12. Withers	22. Forearm	32. Flank
3. Face	13. Chine	23. Knee	33. Upper thigh
4. Muzzle	14. Loin	24. Cannon	34. Stifle
5. Nostril	15. Rump	25. Fetlock	35. Hock
6. Ear	16. Tailhead	26. Pastern	
7. Throat	17. Tail	27. Hoof	
8. Shoulder	18. Pin	28. Dewclaw	
9. Dewlap	19. Switch	29. Milk veins	
10. Brisket	20. Elbow	30. Udder	

Now that we have reviewed the anatomical names for common body parts, we can make use of directional terms to explain where one structure is located relative to another. Only instead of using north, south, east, and west as descriptors, we use the following medical jargon: (1, 3, 4, 6–8)

- Cranial vs. caudal

  - Cranial means towards the patient's head, whereas caudal means towards the patient's tail
  - examples:

    The shoulder is cranial to the flank.
    The flank is caudal to the shoulder.

- Deep vs. superficial

    - Deep means further from the surface, whereas superficial means closer to the surface
    - examples:

        The dermis is deep to the epidermis.
        The epidermis is superficial to the dermis.

- Distal vs. proximal

    - Distal means further from the origination of a structure, such as a limb, whereas proximal means nearer to the origination of a structure
    - examples:

        The pastern is distal to the fetlock.
        The fetlock is proximal to the pastern.

- Dorsal vs. ventral

    - Dorsal means towards the back of the patient, whereas ventral means towards the belly of the patient
    - examples:

        The rectum is dorsal to the urinary bladder.
        The urinary bladder is ventral to the rectum.

- Ipsilateral vs. contralateral

    - Ipsilateral refers to the same side, whereas contralateral refers to the opposite side.
    - examples:

        Hemiparesis refers to the weakness of ipsilateral limbs.
        The patient's right eye is ulcerated; the contralateral eye is not.

- Lateral vs. medial

    - lateral means away from midline, whereas medial means towards midline.
    - examples:

        The fifth digit of the cat's forepaw is lateral to the second digit.
        The second digit of the cat's forepaw is medial to the fifth digit.

- Palmar/plantar

    - Palmar/plantar refers to the sole of the foot. Hence, plantigrade refers to an abnormal stance in which a patient's toes and metatarsals are flat and flush against the ground.

- example:

  The digital pads are located on the plantar aspect of each paw.

- Rostral

  - Rostral is more specific than cranial. Rostral means towards the patient's nose.
  - example:

    The philtrum is rostral to the bridge of the nose.

Refer to Figures 2.4 and 2.5 to review these directional terms as they apply to the description of clinical anatomy.

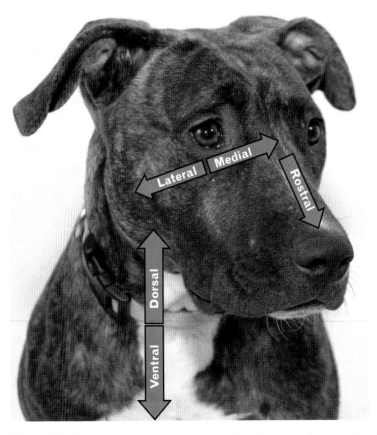

Figure 2.4 Canine external anatomy featuring directional terms. Courtesy of John Schwartz

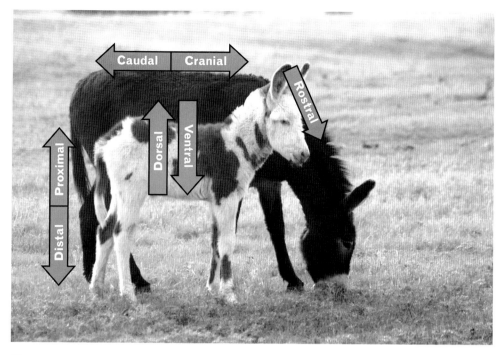

Figure 2.5 Equine external anatomy featuring directional terms. Courtesy of Laura Polerecky

In addition to directional terms, we can describe location of anatomic structures relative to anatomical planes. Anatomical planes refer to hypothetical planes that divide the body into quadrants and in some, but not all, cases, equal halves. (1, 3, 4, 6–8)

The following four primary planes are described in veterinary medicine: (1, 3, 4, 6–8)

- Frontal or dorsal plane
    - parallel to the long axis of the body
    - bisects the body into dorsal and ventral parts

- Median plane
    - bisects the body into equal right and left halves

- Sagittal plane
    - bisects the body into right and left parts

- Transverse plane
    - perpendicular to the long axis of the body
    - bisects the body into cranial and caudal parts.

Refer to Figures 2.6 through 2.8 to review these anatomical planes.

Figure 2.6 Visualizing the anatomical planes using a canine model. The dashed dark grey line represents the median plane. Both dashed light grey lines represent sagittal planes. Courtesy of John Schwartz

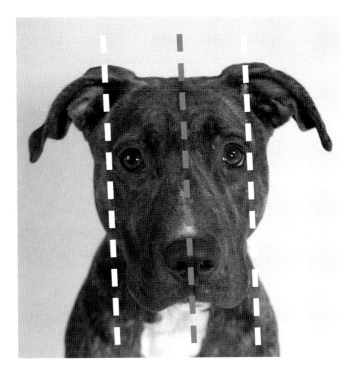

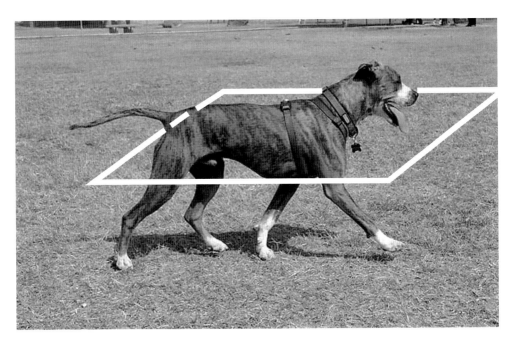

Figure 2.7 Visualizing the frontal or dorsal anatomical plane using a canine model. Courtesy of Analucia Aliaga

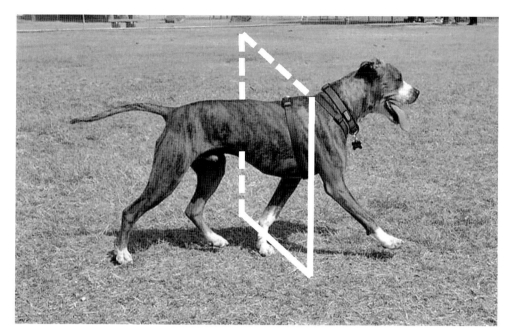

Figure 2.8 Visualizing the transverse anatomical plane using a canine model. Courtesy of Analucia Aliaga

In the same way that an American citizen who speaks only English may feel out of place outside of the United States (U.S.), the language of veterinary medicine may seem like a formidable obstacle.

Medical documentation is rich with jargon. A mastery of medical terms is essential for developing the kind of fluency that is required to document cases accurately. Such fluency is not acquired overnight. It takes time and repetition to overcome the barriers that learning a new language presents.

There are thousands of concepts, definitions, and descriptive terms that comprise veterinary medical vocabulary. From where did these terms originate? Who developed the rules and why do we still follow them?

Nomenclature derived from a central need to ground case discussions in consistent, universally understood dialogue. As early as 1938, the American Veterinary Medical Association (AVMA) prioritized the development of standardized terminology by tasking a committee with establishing veterinary vocabulary.(9) In 1955, the committee published, "Topographic Classification and Etiologic Categories," a veterinary adaptation of the human medical approach, the "Standard Nomenclature of Diseases and Operations" (SNDO).(9, 10) By 1964, this veterinary version was referred to as "Standard Nomenclature of Veterinary Diseases and Operations" (SNVDO).(9, 11)

Both professions shared the same goal: to be able to describe and record physical exam findings and diagnoses without ambiguity.(9, 10, 12–15) As SNDO and SNVDO evolved, specialties within the human medical profession began to expand their vocabularies. For example, the College of American Pathologists published the "Systematized Nomenclature of Pathology" (SNOP) in 1965.(9, 11)

By 1979, SNDO had incorporated such concepts as SNOP into one collective "Systematized Nomenclature for Medicine" (SNOMED).(9) The AVMA followed suit in 1983, unveiling SNOVET.(9) SNOVET was incorporated into SNOMED by 1995.(9) From that point onwards, SNOMED has been the standard for both human and veterinary medicine.(9)

SNOMED continues to evolve with the times. Today, it is referred to as SNOMED-CT, in which "CT" stands for Clinical Terms.(9) The International Health Terminology Standards Development Organization (IHTSDO) is responsible for keeping SNOMED-CT current. (9, 16) SNOMED-CT currently houses more than 300,000 concepts, 800,000 definitions, and 1.3 million relationships.(16) These span the gamut from clinical observations to medical procedures and biological products.(16)

In an effort to pare down the content to make it more accessible and less overwhelming for the veterinary profession, the American Animal Hospital Association (AAHA) and the Veterinary Terminology Service Laboratory (VTSL) at Virginia Polytechnical Institute trimmed SNOMED-CT into AAHA Diagnostic Terms.(9, 17)

In addition, AAHA published a list of standardized abbreviations for veterinary medical documentation to consolidate record-writing and to improve dialogue between primary and referral practices.(18) The list includes commonly used symbols as well as abbreviations for anatomical parts and body regions, physical exam findings, diagnostic tests, and treatment options.(18)

Through standardization, these abbreviations contribute to continuity of care because they can be translated by anyone, even non-veterinary third parties.(18)

Refer to Tables 2.4–2.9 at the end of this chapter to review commonly used, AAHA-approved terms.

AAHA and VTSL were not the only organizations to adopt SNOMED-CT. SNOMED-CT was introduced to the Royal Veterinary College (RVC) Queen Mother Hospital for Animals (QMHA) in 2006.(19, 20) Over the next several years, efforts to refine the system of nomenclature joined forces with those interested in developing a paperless clinical record, the clinical record information system (CRIS).(19, 20) Professor David Church of the RVC and Drs. Ian Ramsey and Jim Anderson of the University of Glasgow Faculty of Veterinary Medicine (UGFVM) took the lead.(19, 20)

From this initiative, the VeNom coding system of veterinary nomenclature was born. (19) This system is maintained by the VeNom Coding Group, which provides codes, free of charge, as an open access resource.(19, 20) Codes are revised quarterly, based upon feedback from end-users.(19, 20)

End-users of the VeNom coding system include, but are not limited to, the: (19, 20)

- Royal (Dick) School of Veterinary Studies
- RVC
- UGFVM
- University of Bristol
- University of Cambridge.

VeNom codes belong to one of several categories: (19, 20)

- Diagnosis
- Presenting complaints
- Procedures

- Therapeutics
- Breeds
- Species.

For ease of use throughout the profession, VeNom coding has been translated into other languages, including German and Spanish.(19, 20)

VeNom coding, SNOMED-CT, and AAHA terminology have been integrated into many electronic practice management systems.(19) This allows for collection of clinical data that can be transferred among the various software platforms.(19)

Table 2.1 Most common prefixes in medical terminology

Prefix	Meaning	Example
a- an-	without	analgesic
ab-	away from	abduction
acantho-	thorn, spine	acanthocyte
acr(o)-	extreme	acromegaly
ad-	towards	adduction
alb-	the color white	albino
allo-	different, other	alloantigen
amph- amphi-	both, on both sides	amphibian
angi-	blood, blood vessel, duct	angiogram
aniso-	not the same; unequal	anisocoria
ankyl(o)-	crooked	ankylosis
ante-	in front of; coming before	antebrachium
arthr- articul(o)-	related to joints	arthroscopy
auto-	pertaining to self	autoimmune
axill-	related to the armpit	axillary
azo-	containing nitrogen	azotemia
bi-	two, double	bilateral
brachy-	short	brachycephalic
brady-	slow	bradycardia
carcin(o)-	cancer-causing	carcinogen
cata-	down, under, against, back	cataract
chemo-	drug	chemotherapy

Table 2.1 *continued*

Prefix	Meaning	Example
circum-	around	circumferential
contra-	against	contraception
cyan(o)-	blue	cyanosis
dacryo-	tears	dacryocystitis
dextro-	right	dextrorotation
dors(i)- dors(o)-	back	dorsiflexion
dys-	bad, ill	dyskinesia
epi-	up, above	epigastric
gamet(o)-	relating to a reproductive cell or unit	gametogenesis
hemi-	half	hemiparesis
hetero-	different	heterogeneous
homo-	same	homogenous
hyper-	above	hypermetria
hypo-	below	hypovolemia
iatr(o)-	relating to medicine or a physician	iatrogenic
inter-	between	interstitial
macro-	large	macrocytosis
mega-	large	megacardia
melan-	dark, black	melanin
micro-	small	microcytosis
neo-	young, new	neonate
oligo-	few	oligospermia
patho-	suffering, disease	pathogen
phlebo-	to gush or overflow	phlebotomist
poly-	many	polyarthritis
pre-	in front of	prescapular
pro-	preceding, in front of	prothrombin
retro-	behind	retro-orbital
tachy-	fast	tachypnea
tetra-	four	tetraparesis
therio-	wild animal, beast	theriogenology
trans-	across, beyond	transplant
uni-	one, alone	unilateral
ventr(o)-	towards the belly	ventral
xen(o)-	foreign	xenobiotic

Table 2.2 Most common roots of body parts and tissues

Body part	Greek root	Latin root
abdomen	lapar-	abdomin-
arm	brachi-	arm-
armpit	----	axill-
back	not-	dors-
bladder	cyst-	vesic-
blood	hem-	sangui-
	hemat-	sanguin-
blood vessel	angi-	vas-
		vasculo-
bone	oste(o)-	ossi-
bone marrow	myel-	medull-
brain	encephal(o)-	cerebr-
breast	mast-	mamm(o)-
cheek	parei-	bucc-
chest	steth-	pector-
ear	ot(o)-	aur(i)-
egg	oo-	ov-
eye	ophthalm(o)-	ocul(o)-
eyelid	blephar(o)-	cili-
		palpebr-
fat	lip(o)-	adip-
finger	dactyl(o)-	digit-
gallbladder	cholecyst(o)-	fell-
gland	aden(o)-	----
glans penis	balon(o)	----
gums	----	gingiv-
hair	trich(o)-	capill-
head	cephal(o)-	capit(o)-
heart	cardi(o)-	cordi-
hip	----	cox-
intestine	enter(o)-	----
jaw	gnath(o)-	----
kidney	nephr(o)-	ren-
lip	cheil(o)-	labi(o)
	chil(o)-	
liver	hepat(o)-	jecor-
loins	episi(o)-	pudend-

Table 2.2 *continued*

Body part	Greek root	Latin root
lungs	pneumon-	pulmo- pulmon(i)-
mouth	stomat(o)-	or-
muscle	my(o)-	----
nail	onych(o)-	ungui-
navel	omphal(o)-	umbilic-
neck	trachel(o)-	cervic-
nose	rhin(o)-	nas-
ovary	oophor(o)-	ovari(o)-
pelvis	pyel(o)-	pelv(i)-
rib	pleur(o)-	cost(o)-
rib cage	thorac(i)- thorac(o)-	----
shoulder	om(o)-	humer(o)-
skin	dermat(o)- derm-	cut- cuticul-
testis	orchi(o)- orchid(o)-	----
throat	pharyng(o)- laryng(o)-	----
toe	dactyl(o)-	digit-
tongue	gloss- glott-	lingu(a)-
tooth	odont(o)-	dent(i)-
tumor	cel- onc(o)-	tum-
urine, urinary system	ur(o)-	urin(o)-
uterus	hyster(o)- metr(o)-	uter(o)-
wrist	carp(o)-	carp-

Table 2.3 Most common suffixes in medical terminology

Suffix	Meaning	Examples
-ac	pertaining to	cardiac
-al		femoral
-ary		biliary
-ic		ophthalmic
-ous		porous
-tic		otic

Suffix	Meaning	Examples
-ad	towards	caudad
-ase	enzyme	amylase
-asthenia	weakness	myasthenia
-ation	process	rotation
-cele	pouching hernia	hydrocele
-centesis	pricking	abdominocentesis
-cidal	killing	bactericidal
-crine	to secrete	endocrine
-dactyl	pertaining to toes	polydactyl
-dipsia	thirst	polydipsia
-dynia	pain	allodynia
-esthesi	sensation	anesthesia
-form	having the shape of	falciform
-genesis	the beginning of something	embryogenesis
-gnosis	knowledge	prognosis
-gram	image record	echocardiogram
-graphy	process of recording	radiography
-iasis	condition of	mydriasis
-itis	inflammation	hepatitis
-lepsy	attack	epilepsy
-lysis	separation	hemolysis
-malacia	softening	chondromalacia
-megaly	enlargement	cardiomegaly
-meter	instrument used to count	pleximeter
-metry	measuring	tonometry
-oid	resembling	sarcoid
-oma	tumor	sarcoma
-opsy	examination	necropsy
-osis	condition or disease	halitosis
-pathy		osteopathy
-penia	deficiency	osteopenia
-pepsia	related to digestion	dyspepsia
-pexy	fixation	gastropexy
-phage -phagia	related to ingestion	copophagia
-phil(ia)	attraction for	neutrophilia

Table 2.3 *continued*

Suffix	Meaning	Examples
-phobia	fear	photophobia
-plasia	formation	hypoplasia
-plegia	paralysis	tetraplegia
-poiesis	production	hematopoiesis
-ptosis	drooping	proptosis
-ptysis	spitting	hemoptysis
-rrhage	bursting	hemorrhage
-rrhaphy	suturing	tarsorrhaphy
-rrhea	flowing	diarrhea
-sclerosis	hardening	atherosclerosis
-scopy	viewing with instrument	otoscopy
-spadias	fissure	hypospadias
-stalsis	contraction	peristalsis
-stasis	stopping	hemostasis
-stenosis	abnormal narrowing	dacryostenosis
-stomy	creating an opening	esophagostomy
-tension	pressure	hypotension
-tome	cutting	osteotome
-tomy	act of cutting	thoracotomy
-tripsy	crushing	neurotripsy
-trophy	development	atrophy
-version	turning	mesioversion
-y	process	surgery

Table 2.4 Commonly used and approved AAHA abbreviations for body parts and regions

Abbreviation	Definition
abd	abdomen
AD	auris dextra, right ear
AS	auris sinistra, left ear
AU	auris uterque, each ear
OD	oculus dexter, right eye
OS	oculus sinister, left eye
OU	oculus uterque, each eye

Table 2.5 Commonly used and approved AAHA abbreviations for diagnoses

Abbreviation	Definition
ARDS	acute respiratory distress syndrome
ARF	acute renal failure
ASD	atrial septal defect
ATE	aortic thromboembolism
BDLD	big dog little dog (trauma)
CRD	chronic renal disease
CRF	chronic renal failure
DDz	dental disease
DM	diabetes mellitus
FAD	flea allergy dermatitis
FB	foreign body
FeLV	feline leukemia virus
FIV	feline immunodeficiency virus
FLUTD	feline lower urinary tract disease
FUO	fever of unknown origin
FUS	feline urological syndrome
Fx	fracture
FxC	closed fracture
FxO	open fracture
GDV	gastric dilatation-volvulus
GSW	gunshot wound
HBC	hit-by-car
HGE	hemorrhagic gastroenteritis
HL	hepatic lipidosis
HOD	hypertrophic cardiomyopathy
HSA	hemangiosarcoma
HWDz	heartworm disease
IBD	inflammatory bowel disease
IMHA	immune-mediated hemolytic anemia
IMTP	immune-mediated thrombocytopenia
IVDD	intervertebral disc disease
KCS	keratoconjunctivitis sicca
LSA	lymphosarcoma
MCT	mast cell tumor
MI	mitral insufficiency
MPL	medial patellar luxation

Table 2.5 *continued*

Abbreviation	Definition
OA	osteoarthritis
Parvo	parvovirus
PLE	protein-losing enteropathy
PLN	protein-losing nephropathy
PRA	progressive retinal atrophy
PRAA	persistent right aortic arch
PSS	portosystemic shunt
Pyelo	pyelonephritis
Pyo	pyometra
RACL	ruptured anterior cruciate ligament
RCCL	ruptured cranial cruciate ligament
UAP	ununited anconeal process
UO	urinary (urethral) obstruction
URI	upper respiratory infection
UTI	urinary tract infection
VAFS	vaccine-associated feline sarcoma
VAS	vaccine-associated sarcoma
VPC	ventricular premature contraction
VSD	ventricular septal defect

Table 2.6 Commonly used and approved AAHA abbreviations for diagnostic tests and treatment options

Abbreviation	Definition
BP	blood pressure
Bx	biopsy
CBC	complete blood cell count
cc	cubic centimeter
Chem	chemistry panel
CRI	constant rate infusion
Euth	euthanize
Glu	glucose
HWT	heartworm test
IC	intracardiac
ID	intradermal
IM	intramuscular
IN	intranasal

Abbreviation	Definition
IO	intraosseous
IP	intraperitoneal
IT	intratracheal
MRI	magnetic resonance imaging
PLR	pupillary light response
PTS	put to sleep
PU	perineal urethrostomy
RTG	ready to go (home)
Rx	prescription
SC	subcutaneous
SG	specific gravity
SQ	subcutaneous
SR	suture removal
STT	Schirmer tear test
Tx	treatment
UA	urinalysis
U cath	urinary catheterization
Vacc/Vx	vaccination

Table 2.7   Commonly used AAHA abbreviations for history and physical examination findings

Abbreviation	Definition
ADR	ain't doing right
BAR	bright, alert, responsive
BARH	bright, alert, responsive, hydrated
BCS	body condition score
BM	bowel movement
BPM	beats per minute
BW	body weight
CRT	capillary refill time
C/S	coughing/sneezing
FS	female spayed
HR	heart rate
LF	left front
LN	lymph node
LPL	left pelvic limb
LR	left rear
LTL	left thoracic limb

Table 2.7 *continued*

Abbreviation	Definition
MN	neutered male
NE	not eating
NED	no evidence of disease
PU/PD	polyuria and polydipsia
QAR	quiet, alert, responsive
QARH	quiet, alert, responsive, hydrated
R	respiration
ROM	range of motion
RPL	right pelvic limb
RR	right rear
RTL	right thoracic limb
T	temperature
TNTC	too numerous to count
TPR	temperature, pulse, and respiration
TTTP	too tense to palpate
V/C/S	vomiting, coughing, and sneezing
V/D	vomiting and diarrhea
WNL	within normal limits

Table 2.8 Commonly used AAHA abbreviations for medical record descriptors

Abbreviation	Definition
CV	cardiovascular
DDx	differential diagnosis
Dx	diagnosis
Dz	disease
EENT	eyes, ears, nose, throat
H/L	heart and lungs
Hx	history
LN	lymph node(s)
MS	musculoskeletal
NS	nervous system
O	owner
PHx	past history
RDVM	referring veterinarian
TC	telephone call
UG	urogenital

Table 2.9 Commonly used and approved AAHA abbreviations for pharmacy

Abbreviation	Definition
Abx	antibiotics
Ad lib	ad libitum, "free choice"
BID	bis in die/twice a day
Bol	bolus
Cap(s)	capsule(s)
EOD	every other day
EOW	every other week
PO	per os/by mouth
PRN	pro re nata/as needed
QD	once daily/every day
QID	four times per day
QOD	every other day
SID	semel in die/once a day
TID	ter in die/three times a day

END-OF-CHAPTER SUMMARY

Veterinary medical documentation is strengthened by using the appropriate jargon, including prefixes, roots, and suffixes to describe:

- body parts
- directional terms
- anatomical planes.

A mastery of veterinary medical jargon facilitates communication about patient care.

To improve dialogue between primary and referral practices, standardized nomenclature has been adopted in the form of SNOMED-CT.

In addition, the American Animal Hospital Association (AAHA) has developed a list of standard abbreviations for use in veterinary medicine. Standard abbreviations exist for medications, medication instructions, body parts and body regions, physical exam findings, diagnostic tests, and treatment options.

Standardized abbreviations allow veterinary medical documentation to be understood, even by non-veterinary professionals.

References

1. Walker-Smith N, Warren E. Veterinary Medical Terminology. Available from: http://www.vspn.org/Library/Misc/VSPN_M02371.htm
2. Romich JA. An Illustrated Guide to Veterinary Medical Terminology. 4th ed. Australia; Stamford, CT: Cengage Learning; 2015. xiv, 642 pp.
3. Taibo A. Veterinary Medical Terminology Guide and Workbook. Ames, Iowa: John Wiley & Sons; 2014.
4. Christenson DE. Veterinary Medical Terminology. 2nd ed. St. Louis, MO: Saunders/Elsevier; 2009. xi, 395 pp.
5. Studdert VP, Gay CC, Blood DC. Saunders Comprehensive Veterinary Dictionary. 4th ed. Edinburgh; New York: Saunders Elsevier; 2012. xiii, 1325 pp.
6. McBride DF. Learning Veterinary Terminology. 2nd ed. St. Louis, MO: Mosby; 2002. xiv, 546 pp.
7. Ehrlich A. Medical Terminology for Health Professions. 8th ed. Clifton Park, NY: Cengage Learning; 2016.
8. Ehrlich A, Schroeder CL. Introduction to Medical Terminology. 3rd ed. Australia; United States: Cengage Learning; 2014. xviii, 478 pp.
9. Zaninelli M, Campagnoli A, Reyes M, Rojas V. The O3-Vet project: integration of a standard nomenclature of clinical terms in a veterinary electronic medical record for veterinary hospitals. Comput Methods Programs Biomed. 2012;108(2):760–772.
10. Thompson ET, Hayden AC. Standard nomenclature of diseases and operations. Hosp Manage. 1954;77(6):37–38; passim.
11. Watson C. SNODOG Glossary Part 1: Introduction, Technical Report. U.S. Department of Energy; 1993.
12. Vermillion CO. Location of tumor diagnoses in a standard nomenclature punched-card disease index. J Am Med Assoc. 1957;165(17):2184–2185.
13. Thompson ET, Slaughter DP. Standard nomenclature in approved cancer clinics. J Am Med Assoc. 1957;163(13):1131–1134.
14. Seasly RH, Brown AF. Disease index for pathology based on standard nomenclature. Am J Clin Pathol. 1957;27(4):429–432.
15. Baron C. The Standard Nomenclature in a general practitioner's office. GP. 1957;16(4):111–112.
16. Shahpori R, Doig C. Systematized Nomenclature of Medicine–Clinical Terms direction and its implications on critical care. J Crit Care. 2010;25(2):364 e1–9.
17. Green JM, editor. The AAHA Diagnostic Terms Subset. Talbot Symposium; 2010; Atlanta, Georgia: American Veterinary Medical Association.
18. AAHA Standard Abbreviations for Veterinary Medical Records. 3rd ed. Lakewood, CO: AAHA Press; 2010.
19. Brodbelt D. Veterinary Nomenclature. Available from: http://www.venomcoding.org/VeNom/Welcome.html
20. Brodbelt D, editor. VeNom Coding. WSAVA/FECAVA/BSAVA World Congress; 2012.

Chapter 3

Structuring the Medical Record

Medical documentation is a broad-sweeping term referring to written notations that establish the provider–patient relationship and support patient care. There are two primary components of medical documentation: administrative and medical record-keeping. The administrative aspect of medical documentation is beyond the scope of this text and is primarily concerned with client registration, contact information, payment history, and insurance carrier. The administrative angle also covers controlled drug and pharmacy logs in addition to financial data for any given practice. By contrast, medical record-keeping is specific to the health history and status of any given patient. Each patient has a unique medical record that tracks the evolution of patient-specific care over time, including familial history, past and present illnesses; examination and diagnostic test reports; major and minor problem lists; therapeutic treatment plans; and responses to treatment.

Veterinary medical records lack standardization in terms of content and format. Although the concept of a medical record is universally understood among veterinarians, veterinary students can attest to the fact that medical records from two distinct practices are more often dissimilar than alike. The disparity is perhaps greatest between the settings of private practice and the teaching hospitals of academic institutions: records trend towards sparse in the former and verbose in the latter.[1] In the author's experience, private practitioners have been known to denounce the academician's tendency to write novel-length case reports; and academicians have been known to censure the practitioner's obsession with brevity. Each group is quick to criticize the other's approach, yet neither group is without the need for self-reflection and improvement.[1, 2] Writing more or writing less is not the solution. Emphasizing efficiency is.[2] Efficiency means prioritizing the clinical needs of the patient without becoming so bogged down in irrelevant details that are included only for the sake of countering the potential for legal action.[2]

3.1 Prioritizing Medical Record Content

There is no universal standard in the veterinary profession that dictates which information must be included in the medical record.(1) Veterinary educators must rely upon accrediting or other overseeing bodies for guidance as to what to instruct, and veterinary graduates must rely upon laws within their practice's jurisdiction to understand what they are legally responsible for including.

The United Kingdom (U.K.)

Within the United Kingdom (U.K.), the Royal College of Veterinary Surgeons (RCVS) regulates all registered veterinary technicians – so-called veterinary nurses – and all veterinarians – so-called veterinary surgeons.(3)

Because the veterinary profession is a self-governing profession within the U.K., the RCVS Council is made up of veterinary surgeons. The RCVS Council seats 42 members. These members include: (3, 4)

- 24 elected veterinary surgeons
- Two members appointed by each university with a veterinary school

  - University of Bristol
  - University of Cambridge
  - University of Edinburgh
  - University of Glasgow
  - University of Liverpool
  - University of London
  - University of Nottingham

- Four members appointed by the Privy Council.

The Privy Council is a formalized group of officials that advises the Sovereign of the U.K.(5)

Collectively, the RCVS is responsible for maintaining codes of conduct that guide the behavior of veterinary professionals.(3, 4)

In addition to regulating veterinary behavior, the RCVS supports legal statutes that relate to the supply, acquisition, storage, prescription, and destruction of pharmaceutical agents.(6)

There is overlap between the codes of conduct as outlined by the RCVS and the Veterinary Medicines Directorate, which is the legal arm of the government that inspects practices and ensures that practicing veterinary surgeons comply with the law.(7)

The Veterinary Medicines Directorate has outlined Veterinary Medicines Regulations (VMRs) that pertain to record-keeping concerning pharmaceutical data.(8, 9) VMRs dictate how medications are to be recorded, both in terms of their supply and administration.(8, 9) Of particular interest are food-producing animals, which, in accordance with European legislation, include horses. Farmers and animal caretakers must maintain medication records on any animal that could enter the food chain for at least five years. (8, 9)

Veterinary surgeons must take care to include the following in so-called medicines records: (9)

- Clinician's name
- Name of product
- Product's batch number
- Administration date
- Amount of product that was administered
- To whom the product was administered
- Withdrawal period, for food-producing animals.

If and when animal caretakers administer pharmaceuticals, they must record all of the above except the clinician's name and the product's batch number.(9) In addition, they must retain proof of purchase for all veterinary medicines and document the following: (9)

- Name of product
- Product's batch number
- Date of purchase
- Amount purchased
- Supplier's name and address.

Product disposal must also be recorded, including how and where the drug was disposed.(9)

Although VMRs are specific in terms of what to document, they do not stipulate how to document.(9) A number of organizations have developed publications that assist with record-keeping to help those involved with animal care be compliant. These publications include: (9)

- Animal Health Distributors Association (AHDA)
- British Beekeepers Association (BBKA)
- The Fish Health Inspectorate
- National Office of Animal Health (NOAH)
- The Pig Veterinary Society.

Individuals may also create their own system. Refer to Figure 3.1 for a sample log for product administration.

In addition to ensuring that documentation concerning pharmaceuticals is accurate and current, RCVS stipulates what constitutes a complete medical record. In accordance with Chapter 13 of the Code of Professional Conduct for Veterinary Surgeons, all patient records must include the following details: (10)

- Examination date
- Examination findings
- Procedures performed

NAME OF PERSON KEEPING RECORD:

ADDRESS: **TELEPHONE NUMBER:**   **FLOCK/HERD NUMBER:**

                              EMAIL:

Date that medication was administered	Patient(s) treated	Name of product that was administered	Batch Number of product that was administered	Date when treatment ended	Date when withdrawal period ended	How much product was administered?	Who administered the product?	Reason for treatment

Figure 3.1 Sample form for record-keeping for product administration

- Diagnostic test results

  - diagnostic imaging
  - labwork

- Preliminary or definitive diagnoses
- Client communication
- Treatment plan

  - therapeutic approach, including prescribed medications
  - management approach to treatment, including an outline for proposed follow-up

- Estimate(s) for veterinary care
- Documentation of client consent
- Documentation when consent is withheld.

Telephone conservations must also be documented, as well as client contact information.(10)

Additional guidelines are provided by organizations such as the British Veterinary Association (BVA) and British Small Animal Veterinary Association (BSAVA). Organizational membership is required to gain access to these materials.

Canada

Within Canada, medical records are considered legal documents. The primary governing body for the profession, the Canadian Veterinary Medical Association (CVMA), stipulates that the following items must be included within the patient record: (11)

- Attending veterinarian's initials
- Client contact information
- Patient name
- Patient identification

  - physical description of patient, including distinguishing features

    - cropped ears
    - dewclaws
    - docked tails
    - scars
    - tattoos

  - signalment: age, sex, sexual status, breed, and species

    - note that mixed breeds should be defined further by weight and height

- Patient history
- Physical examination findings, including patient behavior and mentation
- Diagnostic test results
- Daily updates on hospitalized patients.

In addition to requirements outlined by the CVMA, practicing veterinarians are subject to provincial regulations.

Refer to each province's regulatory body for additional details. For example, the College of Veterinarians of Ontario (CVO) establishes practice standards for the province of Ontario.(12)

The United States (U.S.)

Within the United States (U.S.), state-specific laws including, but not limited to, Veterinary Practice Acts, set the bar in terms of acceptable versus unacceptable documentation. (1, 13) In some cases, state boards of veterinary medical examiners also adopt regulations that practicing veterinarians must follow.(1, 13) These laws and regulations pertain to what kinds of information must be included in the veterinary medical record, and for how long the veterinarian is responsible for maintaining those records.(1, 13)

For example, the state of Florida requires that the following information be included in the medical record of every patient: (14)

- Client name
- Patient identification
- Date of service
- Service performed
- Patient history
- Patient weight, temperature, pulse, and respiration
- Physical examination findings
- Record of any vaccinations that were administered
- Provisional diagnosis.

Note that this constitutes the minimum standard.(1)

The burden falls upon the veterinarian to determine the minimum requirements of the state in which s/he practices.(1) The law should always be consulted before implementing a record system to ensure that standards are met.(1)

Note that state laws and regulations are not limited to record content. They also apply to record retention by the practice.(15) Some state practice acts also have specific requirements regarding the time frame in which veterinarians are expected to follow through with client requests for copies of the medical record.(1)

To encourage national standardization within the United States, the American Animal Hospital Association (AAHA) provides AAHA-accredited hospitals with a series of requirements for medical records.(1, 16) However, these requirements are in addition to those which are required by law.

In most cases, AAHA standards for medical record-keeping exceed the minimum requirements of the states.(1, 16)

3.2 Paper vs. Electronic Record-Keeping

There is no one right way to structure a medical record.

All practitioners develop their own preferences. These preferences may also be shaped by individual practice protocols.

Practice software may also dictate how medical records are structured. For instance, practices that operate in the absence of electronic practice management software have to rely upon paper records. For these to be effective and efficient, they must be structured in a way that achieves a logical flow of information. Information must be easily accessible.

Medium- and large-sized practices are more likely to use electronic medical records (EMRs).(17) The structure of EMRs is based upon the software and the licensing agreement that the individual practice has purchased.

The following are examples of veterinary software, the license to which can be purchased to facilitate all areas of practice management, including record keeping:

- AVImark
- Cornerstone Practice Management
- eVetPractice.com (SERG Solutions)
- ezVet
- Hippo Manager
- Infinity (ImproMed)
- Onward Vet©
- Universal Veterinary Information System (UVIS).

Practice management software and EMRs are relatively new to the veterinary profession. Not all clinicians have had the opportunity to experience EMRs for themselves, and in fact, many still prefer paper records.(17–20)

Cost is frequently cited as an obstacle to the adoption of EMRs by veterinarians, particularly those employed by smaller practices.(17, 18, 21, 22) Additional barriers to EMRs in healthcare include reluctance to adapt to technology; anticipated technological difficulties; perceived time constraints associated with data input; and perceived lack of user-friendly platforms.(17, 18, 23, 24)

On the other hand, EMRs are able to integrate data from one or more clinicians and one or more practices in a way that streamlines communication and reduces medical errors.(25–27) In human healthcare within the U.S. alone, medical errors account for 44,000 deaths per year.(28) These errors cost the healthcare industry an estimated $17 billion annually, not to mention the additional cost to society.(28) To reduce these errors, the U.S. National Academy of Medicine, formerly called the Institute of Medicine, supports the adoption of EMRs. EMRs are thought to more effectively capture, manage, and store patient data.(25, 29) When patient data is managed effectively, medical errors are less likely to occur.

EMRs also facilitate a checks and balances approach to the practice of medicine by detecting adverse health events,(30) flagging prescription errors,(26, 31) and reducing redundancy in diagnostic testing.(32) It is assumed that veterinary practices can capitalize on these same benefits.(17, 20, 23, 24, 33)

Additionally, EMRs serve as a medical database from which patient-specific data can be mined to establish incidence and prevalence of disease within a population.(25) The results of data mining are publishable. These publications can track trends in disease as well as best practices. For instance, retrospective studies may identify the most common surgical complications within a subset of the population or establish the dosing range for medications and anesthetic agents that carries the least amount of adverse events.

Using EMRs as databases for disease is currently underutilized in veterinary medicine. If that were to change, consider the implications that this might have for the veterinary industry. Nearly two thirds of infectious human pathogens are zoonotic.(17, 34) From a public health standpoint alone, improvements in animal disease surveillance are indicated as a safeguard against emerging infectious diseases. The mining of EMRs for data that can propel research forward is an obvious first step towards a better understanding of animal diseases, particularly those that impact human health.(17)

Unfortunately, without financial support or government mandates that require their adoption, veterinary EMRs remain highly variable in terms of content, quality, and capabilities.(35)

An additional concern is that human healthcare software is not necessarily compatible with systems that are currently employed in veterinary practice. So although human healthcare benefits from the EMR's ability to integrate information and streamline hospital flow, veterinary medicine has infrequently experienced these advantages.(24)

3.3 Prioritizing the Structure of the Medical Record

Whether paper-based or electronic, the medical record tends to fit one of three structures:

- Source-oriented approach
- Problem-oriented approach
- Combined approach.

Source-oriented record-keeping is a traditional approach to the medical record. It groups data based upon how data is obtained.(1, 36, 37) For example, patient visit summaries are grouped together. So, too, are clinical pathology reports. Groupings are chronological, and typically present the most current data last.

By contrast, problem-oriented records group data chronologically by clinical problem.(1, 36) For example, if a veterinary patient presented for vomiting, diarrhea, and hematuria, data would be grouped where it is most relevant. For example, every item of the medical record that pertained to hematuria would be lumped together, including:

- The urinary history

  - frequency of urination
  - perceived ease of urination

    - the presence or absence of straining to urinate
    - the presence or absence of vocalizations during urination

  - volume of urine produced

- Urinary tract-specific physical examination findings

  - evaluation of external genitalia
  - urinary bladder palpation
  - rectal palpation of the prostate in male patients

- Urinalysis results

  - urine color
  - urine turbidity
  - urine specific gravity (USG)
  - urine dipstick
  - microscopic evaluation of urine sediment

- Radiographic and/or ultrasonographic findings specific to the urinary tract

  - the presence or absence of nephroliths
  - the presence or absence of ureteroliths
  - the presence or absence of urethral or cystic calculi.

Likewise, relevant data would be grouped under the presenting complaint of vomiting and diarrhea. Because the differential diagnoses for vomiting and diarrhea overlap, the data is likely to fall into more than one category. This repetition may assist the clinician with identifying patterns and trends. As each clinical case is mapped by problem, the clinician is able to see where and how patient problems may be interrelated.

The problem-oriented approach is increasing in popularity as a means of record-keeping because its contents are easier to retrieve. Everything related to clinical problem "x" can be found in one location within the medical record. This is especially helpful for veterinary students and new graduates who may benefit from working through each individual aspect of a multi-layered case, piecemeal.(1, 36)

A combined approach blends source- and problem-oriented record-keeping. This allows clinicians to select aspects of each that maximize efficiency in their practice of veterinary medicine.(1)

3.4 The Problem-Oriented Medical Record (POMR)

The concept of the problem-oriented medical record (POMR) was developed by Lawrence Weed, a medical doctor, in the 1960s.(38–40) In his opinion, the then current system led to "such a tangle of illogically grouped bits of information . . . that one cannot reliably discern how (or if) the physician defined and logically pursued each problem."(38)

Weed expanded upon what he felt to be one of the system's primary shortcomings:

> At present the physician has to read the entire record (often illegible and handwritten) and then sort the data in his mind if he is to know all the patient's difficulties and the extent to which each has been analyzed. There is no evidence that he does this reliably and consistently; he and others using the record lose their way, and problems get neglected, missed entirely or treated out of context.
>
> (38)

It concerned Weed that patient data often became buried in a sea of narrative reports. (38, 39) Hidden from view, this data was lost to follow-up. Patient problems persisted, only to be addressed when and if they flared up. This led to a significant delay in treatment. By the time treatment was initiated, problems that may have been resolved easily at the start could have developed into ailments that were far more insidious.

To reduce lapses in patient care, Weed proposed restructuring the medical record around each clinical problem.(38) The summation of all clinical problems became the patient's problem list. The problem list was not static: it represented a single snapshot in time. As problems resolved, persisted, or intensified, the list required updates. In other words, the problem list became a visual tally of what was going on with the patient, for how long, and with what other ailments concurrently.

Critics of this approach argued that it was too time-consuming but Weed maintained that the start-up time was well worth the investment. What time he lost in set-up, he regained by not having to sift through disorganized data.(38)

An additional benefit of the POMR is that it re-established context by putting patient problems in perspective, relative to one another. In the medical profession, patients rarely present for one problem in isolation.(38) More often than not, there is overlap between problems and/or problems interrelate. Treatment of one problem may occur at the expense of another if problems are considered separately. For example, heart failure and renal disease often occur simultaneously.(38) Historically, medical management of the former has often occurred at the expense of the latter and vice versa because each patient concern is treated as a standalone, separate entity.(38) If patient care is to be effective, it must consider the overarching impact of treatment. Treatment for the heart must be considered in light of renal health, and treatment of renal disease must be considered in light of cardiac health. Weed's POMR encouraged clinicians to identify links between problems and to consider the patient as a whole entity rather than its individual parts.(38)

In addition to linking problems to one another, Weed wanted to link knowledge across medical disciplines. In his opinion:

Real problems always cross specialties. If a patient has chest pain, it could be a cardiovascular problem. It could be a lung problem. It could be a spine problem. They could have a broken rib. There can be a hundred causes of chest pain. Well, when a patient goes to see a cardiologist, can she be sure that he *knows* the symptoms and findings of a thoracic disk [herniation], that doesn't have anything to do with her heart?(40)

Weed believed that integration of medical knowledge across disciplines was essential for high-quality patient care, yet specialty practice at times handicapped clinicians' ability to be thorough.(40) From his perspective, it seemed that some specialists wore blinders. He postulated that these experts had worked for so long in such a narrow field that they had forgotten what else *other than* their specialty could be plaguing their patients. (40) There was simply too much for any human mind to learn and process. Human medicine was evolving as a field faster than doctors could keep up with the knowledge base. Weed hoped that POMR would evolve into a computer-based system that could fill in those gaps for specialists and encourage critical thinking in areas outside of their forte.(40)

Although the technological support for this computer-based system fell short, the concept of POMR took off. As Medical Director, Weed first introduced POMR into his teaching institution, the Eastern Maine General Hospital.(39) One of his graduating interns, Harold Cross, pitched the concept to private practice.(39) Subsequent buy-in by human medical educators, such as Willis Hurst, led to the adoption of POMR by thousands of physicians across the globe.(39)

In the early 1970s, the POMR was adapted for use in veterinary medicine by educators at the University of Georgia's veterinary teaching hospital.(41) Thereafter, most veterinary colleges in North America accepted the POMR as the standard for record-keeping.(41)

Although different versions exist to meet the needs of the institution and its employees, the basic framework of the POMR involves four structurally distinct sections: (1, 42)

* A patient profile or database
* A current and actively evolving problem list

    * each clinical problem is listed
    * the date of onset for each clinical problem is listed
    * the date when each clinical problem resolved is listed
    * any item that has yet to be resolved remains on the list as an active problem

* A visit summary
* A problem-oriented patient plan.

Collectively, these four sections present a logical flow to case management.(41) When a patient first presents for evaluation, a patient-specific database is collected. This data allows the veterinarian to identify one or more patient-specific problems based upon the history and physical examination findings. A visit summary tasks the clinician to consider how clinical problems may interrelate as well as the best course of action for proceeding with patient care. Treatment is then initiated as part of the patient's management plan. The veterinarian contracts with the client to return to the clinic at pre-determined intervals to reassess the patient. The patient's response to treatment is noted, and the plan is amended accordingly.(41)

3.5 The Patient Profile or Database

The patient profile or database refers to all patient data, including, but not limited to:

* Signalment
* Previous medical history, including past diagnoses
* Current medical history, including active problems and new concerns.

This data is important for establishing a baseline and tracking the progress of a patient over time.(41)

Note that there is not one "right" approach to data collection. The contents of a patient database are likely to vary between practices, based upon individual practice needs.

Most databases include a comprehensive patient history and pertinent findings from the patient's physical examination.(41) Beyond that, there is intense disagreement as to what constitutes a minimum database.(38)

As a veterinary student, I was taught that every minimum database includes a complete blood count (CBC), chemistry panel, and urinalysis (UA). Some colleagues at other institutions include imaging as part of their minimum database. Others prioritize serological status.

There is logic to the concept of a minimum database, particularly within multi-doctor practices. It encourages clinicians to share a similar approach to case management and to provide an equivalent level of care.(43)

However, practices must weigh the need for standardization against financial factors, such as client cost, and what is in the best interest of the patient.(43) Which diagnostic tests are essential to *every* patient? Which are essential for *select* patients? Should certain tests be prioritized? If so, do tests take priority always or only under certain circumstances? What, if any, are the exceptions to the rules?

Evidence-based clear-cut guidelines for when to test which patient and for which diseases are hard to come by in the veterinary medical literature.(44–51) Therefore, organizations such as AAHA are moving away from the one-size-fits-all patient database. Instead, they are leaning towards a patient-specific approach. That is, recommendations for diagnostic testing are tailored to the patient.(52)

3.6 The Problem List

The problem list is a dynamic record of clinical signs and their associated diagnoses.(38) Consider it to be a living, breathing table of contents for each patient's medical record. (38) It provides a continuous update of patient problems, and allows anyone within the veterinary team to distinguish between active and inactive issues on a cursory glance.(38)

Refer to Figures 3.2 and 3.3 for sample blank and completed problem lists.

Just as patient health evolves, so, too, does the problem list. In the initial stages of the work-up, prior to diagnostic intervention, patient problems are often poorly understood and therefore can only be vaguely defined.(38, 53) For example, the following patient problems are described at an appropriate level of understanding for a patient that is in the initial phase of assessment:

- Abdominal pain
- Dyspnea
- Dysuria
- Forelimb lameness
- Halitosis
- Pruritus
- Scooting.

As the work-up proceeds and diagnostic interventions provide additional insight into patient health status, the clinician progressively understands more about the case. The problem list should reflect this knowledge gain. Because the problem list is not static, its contents can be clarified to reflect the clinician's current level of understanding.(38, 53)

Consider the same examples as above and how these may be refined based upon additional information that has been provided by a comprehensive patient work-up:

- Abdominal pain
  - stomach pain
- Dyspnea
  - upper airway obstruction
- Dysuria
  - feline lower urinary tract disease
- Forelimb lameness
  - ununited anconeal process (UAP) of the right elbow
- Halitosis
  - grade 2 periodontal disease
- Pruritus
  - demodicosis
- Scooting
  - anal sacculitis.

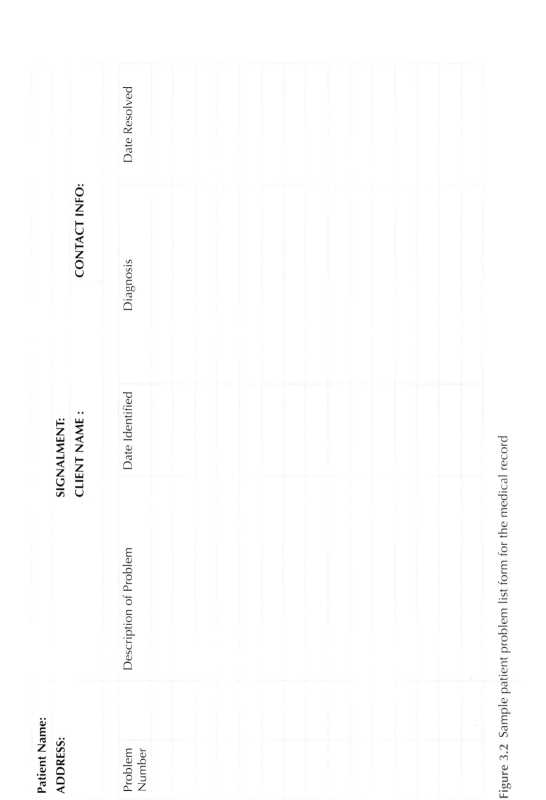

Figure 3.2 Sample patient problem list form for the medical record

Patient Name: BAILEY ENGLAR

ADDRESS:
xxxxxxxxxxxxxxxxxxxxxxxxxxxxx
Xxxxxxxxxxxxxxxxxxxxxxxxxxxx

Signalment: 13-year-old Female Spayed (FS) Tonkinese cat

CLIENT NAME: Ryane Englar   **CONTACT INFO: xxxxxxxxxxxxxxxxx**

Problem Number	Description of Problem	Date Identified	Diagnosis	Date Resolved
1	Intermittent orofacial tic	3/20/18	Feline Orofacial Pain Syndrome (FOPS) (Presumptive)	Under treatment
2	Overdue on rabies vaccination	3/28/18	Incomplete Patient Database	Ongoing
3	Overdue on FVRCP vaccination	3/28/18	Incomplete Patient Database	Ongoing
4	Ceruminous aural discharge AD	3/28/18	Otitis externa AD (Definitive)	Under treatment
5	Loss of balance	3/29/18	Otitis media AU (Definitive)	Under treatment
6	High-end normal blood urea nitrogen (BUN): 30 (15-31mg/dL)	3/28/18	Renal Insufficiency (Definitive)	Under treatment
7	High-end normal creatinine: 1.8 (0.9-1.9mg/dL)	3/28/18	Renal Insufficiency (Definitive)	Under treatment
8	Low urine specific gravity (USG) 1.013	3/28/18	Renal Insufficiency (Definitive)	Under treatment
9	Fractured right maxillary canine tooth	3/28/18	Complicated Root Fracture (Definitive)	3/29/18 (surgically extracted)
10	Subgingival mass adjacent to left mandibular canine tooth	3/28/18	Salivary gland obstruction / mineralization (Definitive)	3/29/18 (surgically excised)
11	Subgingival mass adjacent to right mandibular canine tooth	3/28/18	Salivary gland obstruction / mineralization (Definitive)	3/29/18 (surgically excised)

Figure 3.3 Completed sample patient problem list form for the medical record

This funnel approach – starting out broadly, and then narrowing down the diagnosis – minimizes the tunnel vision that might occur if clinicians tried to define problems too quickly, without supporting evidence.

For example, if *stomach pain* were listed instead of *abdominal pain* in the early stages of the work-up, the clinician would be far less likely to consider other sources of abdominal pain. Colitis may be overlooked as a possibility because the veterinarian has already led himself to believe that the source of the pain is definitively the stomach. But what if the pain were, in fact, related to a splenic mass? The potential for a splenic mass to occur may not even be on the veterinarian's radar because only the stomach was considered. The patient may have been sent home erroneously with a script for antacids when in fact what the patient needed was diagnostic imaging.

Another example pertains to *forelimb lameness*. If *elbow pain* was listed instead of *forelimb lameness*, then the clinician may overlook a shoulder injury that is in fact responsible for the presenting complaint.

At the same time, one must be cautious not to understate a problem.(53) Being too broad can also obstruct decision-making and prevent the clinician from unearthing a diagnosis.(53)

For example, listing *breathing issue* is not specific enough. *Breathing issue* could include virtually any abnormality from the nares to the mechanical action of the diaphragm. Documenting *increased expiratory effort* would be more beneficial. This phrase at least narrows down the act of breathing to the portion of the respiratory cycle that is involved.

3.7 Introduction to SOAP Notes

SOAP notes are structured written summaries of patient encounters.(54) These include new patient visits, problem-specific consultations ("sick visits"), recheck appointments, referrals, second opinions, and inpatient care such as medical boarding, hospitalization, anesthetic or surgical procedures.

SOAP notes facilitate healthcare communication by structuring case visits so that: (54)

1. Case details may be summarized concisely
2. Case details may be recalled accurately
3. Patient problems can be addressed systematically
4. Patient problems can be followed up
5. Members of the veterinary team can understand the rationale for patient care
6. Members of the veterinary team can follow the progression of patient care.

The SOAP note consists of four components: (54–58)

- "S" for Subjective
- "O" for Objective
- "A" for Assessment
- "P" for Plan.

For some students, it is helpful to consider that the SOAP note segregates information based upon who provided it. For example, the "S" in SOAP groups data that is most typically provided by the veterinary client, whereas the "O," "A," and "P" group data that is provided primarily by the veterinary team.(58)

END-OF-CHAPTER SUMMARY

There is no universal standard in veterinary medicine that dictates what to include in the medical record.

* Veterinary educators look to accrediting bodies for guidance
* Veterinary graduates adhere to guidelines from their practice's jurisdiction.

Medical records may be paper-based or electronic, and their structure varies:

* Source-oriented
* Problem-oriented
* Combination approach.

The concept of the problem-oriented medical record (POMR) was developed by Lawrence Weed in the 1960s in order to:

* Create a systematic approach to documentation
* Improve continuity of care and transfer of care
* Establish a context for the patient's current situation
* Interrelate the patient's presenting complaints
* Link knowledge across medical disciplines.

The POMR was adapted for use in veterinary medicine in the early 1970s and can be divided into four sections:

* Patient profile or database
* Problem list
* Visit summary
* Problem-oriented plans.

The visit summary takes the form of a SOAP note, in which:

* "S" stands for Subjective
* "O" stands for Objective
* "A" stands for Assessment
* "P" stands for Plan.

References

1. Wilson JF. Law and Ethics of the Veterinary Profession. Yardley, PA: Priority Press, Ltd.; 2000.
2. Gutheil TG. Fundamentals of medical record documentation. Psychiatry (Edgmont). 2004;1(3): 26–28.
3. RCVS: Setting Veterinary Standards; 2018. Available from: https://www.rcvs.org.uk/home/
4. Who We Are; 2018. Available from: https://www.rcvs.org.uk/who-we-are/
5. Current Reviews: Royal College of Veterinary Surgeons; 2013. Available from: http://www.enqa.eu/index.php/royal-college-of-veterinary-surgeons-rcvs/
6. Veterinary Medicines; 2017. Available from: https://www.rcvs.org.uk/setting-standards/advice-and-guidance/code-of-professional-conduct-for-veterinary-surgeons/supporting-guidance/veterinary-medicines/
7. Veterinary Medicines Directorate; 2018. Available from: https://www.gov.uk/government/organisations/veterinary-medicines-directorate
8. Veterinary Medicines; 2014. Available from: https://www.bva.co.uk/News-campaigns-and-policy/Policy/Medicines/Veterinary-medicines/
9. Record Keeping Requirements for Veterinary Medicinal Products; 2009. Available from: https://www.gov.uk/government/uploads/system/uploads/attachment_data/file/424670/VMGNote14.PDF
10. Clinical and Client Records; 2017. Available from: https://www.rcvs.org.uk/setting-standards/advice-and-guidance/code-of-professional-conduct-for-veterinary-surgeons/supporting-guidance/clinical-and-client-records/
11. Medical Records; 2018. Available from: https://www.canadianveterinarians.net/policy-advocacy/documenting-abuse-medical-records
12. Professional Practice Standards: Medical Records; 2015. Available from: https://cvo.org/CVO/media/College-of-Veterinarians-of-Ontario/Resources%20and%20Publications/Professional%20Practice%20Standards/MedicalRecordsPPS2015.pdf
13. Principles of Veterinary Medical Ethics of the AVMA: American Veterinary Medical Association; [5/30/17]. Available from: https://www.avma.org/kb/policies/pages/principles-of-veterinary-medical-ethics-of-the-avma.aspx
14. West's Florida Statutes Annotated. Title XXXII. Regulation of Professions and Occupations (Chapters 454–493). Chapter 474. Veterinary Medical Practice. Michigan State University; [5/30/17]. Available from: https://www.animallaw.info/statute/fl-veterinary-veterinary-medical-practice
15. Records Retention: American Veterinary Medical Association; 2014. Available from: https://www.avma.org/Advocacy/StateAndLocal/Pages/sr-records-retention.aspx
16. Medical Records Manual. Denver, CO: American Animal Hospital Association; 1978.
17. Krone LM, Brown CM, Lindenmayer JM. Survey of electronic veterinary medical record adoption and use by independent small animal veterinary medical practices in Massachusetts. J Am Vet Med Assoc. 2014;245(3):324–332.
18. Lorenzi NM, Kouroubali A, Detmer DE, Bloomrosen M. How to successfully select and implement electronic health records (EHR) in small ambulatory practice settings. BMC Med Inform Decis Mak. 2009;9:15.
19. McCurdy HD. The paperless practice. J Am Vet Med Assoc. 2001;218(11):1776–1777.
20. Pollari FL, Bonnett BN, Allen DG, Bamsey SC, Martin SW. Quality of computerized medical record abstract data at a veterinary teaching hospital. Prev Vet Med. 1996;27(3–4): 141–154.

21. Simon SR, Kaushal R, Cleary PD, Jenter CA, Volk LA, Poon EG, et al. Correlates of electronic health record adoption in office practices: a statewide survey. J Am Med Inform Assoc. 2007;14(1):110–117.

22. Thakkar M, Davis DC. Risks, barriers, and benefits of EHR systems: a comparative study based on size of hospital. Perspect Health Inf Manag. 2006;3:5.

23. Smith-Akin KA, Bearden CF, Pittenger ST, Bernstam EV. Toward a veterinary informatics research agenda: an analysis of the PubMed-indexed literature. Int J Med Inform. 2007;76(4):306–312.

24. Zaninelli M, Tangorra FM, Castano S, Ferrara A, Ferro E, Brambilla PG, et al. The O3-Vet project: a veterinary electronic patient record based on the web technology and the ADT-IHE actor for veterinary hospitals. Comput Methods Programs Biomed. 2007;87(1):68–77.

25. Lobach DF, Detmer DE. Research challenges for electronic health records. Am J Prev Med. 2007;32(5 Suppl):S104–111.

26. Bates DW, Cohen M, Leape LL, Overhage JM, Shabot MM, Sheridan T. Reducing the frequency of errors in medicine using information technology. J Am Med Inform Assoc. 2001;8(4):299–308.

27. Overhage JM, Tierney WM, Zhou XH, McDonald CJ. A randomized trial of "corollary orders" to prevent errors of omission. J Am Med Inform Assoc. 1997;4(5):364–375.

28. McCullough JS, Casey M, Moscovice I, Prasad S. The effect of health information technology on quality in U.S. hospitals. Health Aff (Millwood). 2010;29(4):647–654.

29. Key Capabilities of an Electronic Health Record System. Washington, DC: Institute of Medicine; 2003.

30. Bates DW, Evans RS, Murff H, Stetson PD, Pizziferri L, Hripcsak G. Detecting adverse events using information technology. J Am Med Inform Assoc. 2003;10(2):115–128.

31. Chung K, Choi YB, Moon S. Toward efficient medication error reduction: error-reducing information management systems. J Med Syst. 2003;27(6):553–560.

32. Bates DW, Kuperman GJ, Rittenberg E, Teich JM, Fiskio J, Ma'luf N, et al. A randomized trial of a computer-based intervention to reduce utilization of redundant laboratory tests. Am J Med. 1999;106(2):144–150.

33. Hornof WJ, Brentson PR, Self JA, Ballance DW. Development of a complete electronic medical record in an academic institution. J Am Vet Med Assoc. 2001;218(11):1771–1775.

34. Taylor LH, Latham SM, Woolhouse ME. Risk factors for human disease emergence. Philos Trans R Soc Lond B Biol Sci. 2001;356(1411):983–989.

35. Allen S. Electronic Health Records in Veterinary Medicine: Why a Tree Kangaroo Might Have a Better Electronic Medical Record Than You Do. IEEE Pulse. January/February 2017. Available from: https://pulse.embs.org/january-2017/electronic-health-records-veterinary-medicine/.

36. Hayrinen K, Saranto K, Nykanen P. Definition, structure, content, use and impacts of electronic health records: a review of the research literature. Int J Med Inform. 2008;77(5):291–304.

37. Tange HJ, Hasman A, de Vries Robbe PF, Schouten HC. Medical narratives in electronic medical records. Int J Med Inform. 1997;46(1):7–29.

38. Weed LL. Medical records that guide and teach. N Engl J Med. 1968;278(11):593–600.

39. Jacobs L. Interview with Lawrence Weed, MD–the father of the problem-oriented medical record looks ahead. Perm J. 2009;13(3):84–89.

40. Wright A, Sittig DF, McGowan J, Ash JS, Weed LL. Bringing science to medicine: an interview with Larry Weed, inventor of the problem-oriented medical record. J Am Med Inform Assoc. 2014;21(6):964–968.

41. Lorenz MD, Neer TM, Demars PL. Small Animal Medical Diagnosis. 3rd ed. Ames, Iowa: Wiley-Blackwell; 2009. xv, 502 pp.

42. Weed LL. Shedding our illusions: a better way of medicine. Fertil Steril. 2004;81 Suppl 2:45–52.

43. Kipperman BS. The demise of the minimum database. J Am Vet Med Assoc. 2014;244(12):1368–1370.

44. Fleming JM, Creevy KE, Promislow DE. Mortality in North American dogs from 1984 to 2004: an investigation into age-, size-, and breed-related causes of death. J Vet Intern Med. 2011;25(2):187–198.

45. Lund EM, Armstrong PJ, Kirk CA, Kolar LM, Klausner JS. Health status and population characteristics of dogs and cats examined at private veterinary practices in the United States. Am Vet Med Assoc. 1999;214(9):1336–1341.

46. Bartlett PC, Van Buren JW, Neterer M, Zhou C. Disease surveillance and referral bias in the veterinary medical database. Prev Vet Med. 2010;94(3-4):264–271.

47. Guptill L, Glickman L, Glickman N. Time trends and risk factors for diabetes mellitus in dogs: analysis of veterinary medical data base records (1970–1999). Vet J. 2003;165(3):240–247.

48. Glickman LT, Moore GE, Glickman NW, Caldanaro RJ, Aucoin D, Lewis HB. Purdue University–Banfield National Companion Animal Surveillance Program for emerging and zoonotic diseases. Vector Borne Zoonotic Dis. 2006;6(1):14–23.

49. Vogt AH, Rodan I, Brown M, Brown S, Buffington CA, Forman MJ, et al. AAFP-AAHA: Feline life stage guidelines. J Am Anim Hosp Assoc. 2010;46(1):70–85.

50. Pittari J, Rodan I, Beekman G, Gunn-Moore D, Polzin D, Taboada J, et al. American Association of Feline Practitioners. Senior care guidelines. J Feline Med Surg. 2009;11(9):763–778.

51. Senior Care Guidelines Task Force, Epstein M, Kuehn NF, Landsberg G, Lascelles BD, Marks SL, et al. AAHA senior care guidelines for dogs and cats. J Am Anim Hosp Assoc. 2005;41(2):81–91.

52. Bartges J, Boynton B, Vogt AH, Krauter E, Lambrecht K, Svec R, et al. AAHA canine life stage guidelines. J Am Anim Hosp Assoc. 2012;48(1):1–11.

53. Lane I. The Problem Oriented Medical Approach. Available from: http://libguides.utk.edu/ld.php?content_id=7167021

54. Cameron S, Turtle-song I. Learning to write case notes using the SOAP format. J Couns Dev. 2002;80(3):286–292.

55. Rockett J, Lattanzio C, Christensen C. The Veterinary Technician's Guide to Writing SOAPS: A Workbook for Critical Thinking. Heyburn, Idaho: Rockett House Publishing LLC; 2013.

56. Borcherding S. Documentation Manual for Writing SOAP Notes in Occupational Therapy. 2nd ed. Thorofare, NJ: SLACK Incorporated; 2005.

57. Kettenbach G. Writing Patient/Client Notes: Ensuring Accuracy in Documentation. 4th ed. Philadelphia: F.A. Davis Company; 2004. 248 pp.

58. Kettenbach G. Writing SOAP Notes: With Patient/Client Management Formats. 3rd ed. Philadelphia: F.A. Davis Company; 2004.

Chapter 4

The "S" in SOAP Notes

The "S" in SOAP notes stands for *subjective*.(1–5) Subjective data is largely historical and relies heavily upon the veterinary client to describe what s/he has observed, to what degree, in what frequency, and for how long.(1–5)

4.1 Introduction to History-Taking

As the technology in healthcare has evolved, it may be tempting to substitute diagnostics for a comprehensive health history. However, the diagnostic value of history-taking cannot be understated.(6) In fact, it has been said of human medicine that roughly two thirds of diagnoses can be made based upon a comprehensive history alone.(7)

History-taking plays an even greater role in veterinary medicine because veterinary patients cannot speak our language. Veterinarians must rely upon clients to provide insight that will be most productive to the outcome of the consultation.

In a primary care setting, when meeting a new patient for the first time, it is particularly important that history-taking be comprehensive.(8) By contrast, emergency visits require the clinician to prioritize stabilization of the patient over all else.(8) For example, a hit-by-car dog requires immediate medical attention, including, but not limited to:

- Analgesia
- Baseline bloodwork
- Flow-by oxygen
- Imaging studies
- Intravenous (IV) catheterization
- Shock bolus of IV fluids.

In this clinical scenario, history-taking must initially take a back seat to life-saving interventions. It would be inappropriate to question the dog's owner about flea and tick preventative while trying to stabilize the patient. What is urgent is addressed first and saving the patient's life becomes the priority. Ectoparasites can be discussed later, if the patient survives the acute phase of trauma.(8)

Assuming that the patient is stable, a comprehensive history should include: (1–5)

- Demographic data
- Presenting complaint or chief complaint (cc)

    - a concise summary statement that identifies the reason for the veterinary medical consultation

- Client expectations
- Lifestyle
- Activity level
- Travel history
- Serological status
- Diet history

    - meals

        – meal contents
        – meal frequency
        – meal volume

    - treats and table scraps

- Current medications

    - over-the-counter products
    - prescriptions
    - vitamins
    - supplements

- History of preventative care, including vaccinations
- Known familial, medical, surgical, and reproductive history
- Past pertinent diagnostic tests and test results, including laboratory and imaging
- Past pertinent therapeutic trials and outcomes.

4.2 Demographic Data

Demographic data includes the patient's age, sex, sexual status, breed, and species. Specifically, this data constitutes the patient's signalment.

The following are examples of signalment among companion animal patients:

- 8-month-old, female spayed (FS) Ragdoll cat
- 1-year-old, female intact (FI) Chihuahua dog
- 4-year-old, male castrated (MC) Rottweiler dog
- 9-year-old, male intact (MI) Golden Retriever dog
- 12-week-old, FS domestic shorthair (DSH) kitten.

Note that the order of the signalment depends upon the clinician's preference and writing style. Some clinicians prefer to write *intact female* (IF) or *intact male* (IM). Others write *male neutered* (MN) and *female neutered* (FN).

Signalment may also include species-specific terminology. For instance, when defining sex and sexual status:

- An intact male cat is referred to as a tomcat
- An intact female cat is referred to as a queen
- An intact male dog is referred to as a stud
- An intact female dog is referred to as a bitch.

Horses and cows also have unique terminology to describe sex and sexual status:

- An intact male horse is referred to as a stallion
- An intact male of the species, *Bos taurus*, is referred to as a bull
- An intact female horse is referred to as a mare
- An intact female *Bos taurus* is referred to as a cow
- An intact female *Bos taurus* that has not yet had a calf is referred to as a heifer
- A castrated male horse is referred to as a gelding
- A castrated male *Bos taurus* is referred to as a steer.

In addition, demographic data includes regional-specific terminology. For example:

- *DSH* versus *moggie*

  - the DSH cat is one of mixed ancestry, that is, it is said to be the mutt of the feline world
  - in the U.K., a cat of mixed ancestry is sometimes referred to as a moggie

- *Entire* versus *intact*

  - *intact* is a descriptor used in the U.S. to indicate that the patient has not been de-sexed
  - *entire* is a descriptor used more commonly in Europe to indicate that the patient has not been de-sexed.

Demographic data may also include patient identifiers, such as coat color. The base coat colors of companion animals include:

- Black
- Grey
- Blue
- Brown
- Red
- Gold
- Yellow
- Cream
- White.

Breeds often have different names for the same coat colors. For example, Siamese cats are typically referred to by their point coloration pattern:

- Seal point (brown)
- Flame point (red–orange)
- Blue point (grey)
- Lilac point (lavender).

Although Tonkinese cats also have points, they are named distinctly. What looks to be a seal point Tonkinese is actually called champagne mink in color.(9)

Names of coat colors also vary between species. Consider horses, for instance. The most common base coat colors in horses include:

- Bays
- Chestnut
- Grey.

Less common base coat colors in horses include:

- Black
- Buckskin
- Roan
- Cremello
- Dun
- White.

Although coat color identification is beyond the scope of this textbook, it is an important identifying feature to consider including in the medical record.

Other demographic data, such as patient breed, may prove useful in considering the various causes of the presenting complaint, particularly given that many breed predispositions to disease have been established in veterinary medicine.(10)

Examine the samples that have been provided below:

- 1-year-old, female spayed *Maine Coon cat*
- 3-year-old, female intact *Standard poodle dog*
- 5-year-old, male castrated *Miniature schnauzer dog*
- 7-year-old, male intact *Boxer dog*
- 12-week-old, female spayed *DSH.*

Based upon breed alone, I could speculate as to what the patient is being treated for, particularly if each example above was supplemented with the presenting complaint:

- 1-year-old, female spayed Maine Coon cat, presenting for acute collapse and dyspnea
- 3-year-old, female intact Standard poodle dog, presenting for waxing/waning diarrhea
- 5-year-old, male castrated Miniature schnauzer dog, presenting for abdominal pain and vomiting
- 7-year-old, male intact Boxer dog, presenting for dyschezia
- 12-week-old, female spayed DSH, presenting for upper airway congestion.

Based upon breed, sex, sexual status, and presenting complaint, a top differential diagnosis for the Maine Coon cat is hypertrophic cardiomyopathy (HCM).(10–12) Hypoadrenocorticism is a top differential diagnosis for the Standard poodle(13–15); pancreatitis, for the Miniature schnauzer(16, 17); and benign prostatic hypertrophy, for the Boxer(18, 19).(10) Upper respiratory infections (URIs) are common in kittens, particularly those from catteries or local shelters.

It may seem obvious that the presenting complaint should be established through history-taking and subsequently included in the "S" of the SOAP. However, veterinarians may fail to inquire, assuming that the client is here to discuss only that which is written in the schedule. This may or may not be accurate. It may also have changed in the time it took for the patient to re-present for a recheck appointment.

One particular case involving a limping Labrador Retriever dog comes to mind. At the time that the client called to schedule the appointment, the week prior to presentation, the dog was lame in the right pelvic limb. This was documented as the client's chief concern in the appointment ledger. If I had not, as the clinician, clarified this to be true, I may never have tracked the progression of the disease or realized that the dog had since developed shifting leg lameness. Shifting leg lameness brought borreliosis to mind. Although the dog still required an examination on my part to rule out cranial cruciate ligament rupture, infectious disease became a likely differential diagnosis.

4.3 Clarifying Questions and History-Taking

Clarifying questions not only round out the differential diagnosis list, they also help the clinician to gain as much detail as is possible about the presenting complaint. Consider history-taking to be a treasure hunt. Your job as the clinician is to find buried treasure. You cannot find buried treasure if your approach is superficial. You need to dig deep to find the answers you are seeking and to guide the client to provide the level of detail necessary to lead you to a diagnosis.

To be as complete as possible, consider taking a journalist's approach by asking the client the five Ws: (20, 21)

* Who?
* What?
* When?

* Where?
* Why?

Some might expand this set to include a sixth guiding question, how? (20, 21)

For example, let's explore the case of a 3-month-old puppy that presents on emergency for vomiting. Using the journalist's approach, the veterinarian should take care to address the content that is outlined by the following questions:

* Who?

  * Who (else) in the house (if anyone) is vomiting?
  * Who (if anyone) has the puppy been exposed to?

- What?

  - What has the owner observed?
  - What does the vomitus look like?
  - What is the puppy's appetite?
  - What is the puppy's activity level?

- When?

  - When did the vomiting start?
  - When was the last episode of vomiting?
  - When does vomiting occur relative to meal time?

- Where?

  - Where has the puppy been within the past two weeks (i.e. kennel, grooming facility, doggie day care, etc.)?
  - Where has the puppy travelled (i.e. out of state or out of the country)?
  - Where is the puppy from (i.e. a breeder, a pet store, the shelter, etc.)?

- Why?

  - Why does the owner think the puppy is vomiting?

- How?

  - How does the puppy act before, during, and after each episode of vomiting?
  - How are the puppy's bowel movements?
  - How has the puppy's appetite changed?
  - How has the puppy's energy level changed?

Note that this sampling of questions represents a mix of closed- and open-ended questions.

Closed-ended questions are conclusive. They collect data that is easy to quantify because the answers to closed-ended questions are typically short or abbreviated, if not one-word.

Closed-ended questions frequently ask the client to weigh in on a statement with either a definitive *yes* or *no*:

- Has Ginny been sneezing?
- Have you noticed any coughing?
- Is Guinevere using the litter box?
- Is Darwin indoor-only?
- Do you plan on kenneling Dobby?
- Did you notice any blood in Gershwin's urine when he peed in the snow?

Closed-ended questions may also ask the client to respond with a number:

- How many times did Bailey eat yesterday?
- How many times a day does Nina void?

- How many times did Timothy vomit overnight?
- How many times has Bentley been obstructed in the past?

In addition, closed-ended questions may yield answers that come in the form of short phrases, such as, "*What does Pumpkin eat?*" The owner is likely to respond with a brand name or perhaps a description of the bag and/or kibble shape: *the yellow bag with the star-shaped kibble.*

Closed-ended questions have a place in the veterinary consultation: there are instances when the veterinarian requires a definite, cut-and-dry answer. For instance, if a patient is being dropped off at the clinic for surgery under general anesthesia, it is imperative that the clinic ask, "*When did you last feed Ginger?*" Similarly, if a patient codes, it is critical that the veterinarian obtain a *yes* or *no* answer to the question, "*Do you want us to perform CPR on Petey?*"

However, there are limits to the amount of detail that can be obtained by asking closed-ended questions. There are also times during the veterinary consultation when the clinician requires the client to expand upon answers to paint a more complete picture of the presenting complaint.

Consider the patient that presents to the clinic with a history of collapse. The burden falls on the clinician to establish whether the patient's collapse is cardiogenic – due to syncope – versus neurologic – due to seizure. Because most patients have unremarkable physical examinations by the time they present for evaluation, history plays an important part in the diagnostic work-up.(22–30) A description of the event provides a starting point that may raise the veterinarian's index of suspicion to favor one differential diagnosis over the other.

For example, syncope is often preceded by pelvic limb weakness and/or ataxia.(31) These clinical signs occur when cerebral perfusion is reduced, just prior to losing consciousness.(31) When consciousness is lost, it is typically brief.(31) Patients are typically flaccid when they collapse.(31)

On the other hand, seizures have historically been described as having tonic-clonic motor signs, with or without autonomic activity.(31, 32) On average, seizures last longer than syncopal episodes, and patients are typically slower to recover.(31) The post-ictal phase that immediately follows a seizure is often characterized by confusion. This may last minutes to hours. Transient behavioral changes and compromised vision are common during this period.

Asking closed-ended questions to decipher the patient history in such a complex case is going to be challenging. The veterinarian might need to ask dozens of closed-ended questions in order to obtain the level of detail that s/he is seeking:

- Was Juniper acting strange before this episode?
- Did Finnegan appear to be weak in his hind limbs before the episode?
- Did Justin seem wobbly just before the incident?
- How long did the event last?
- Did it take a while for Lowell to recover?

- How long did it take for Lowell to recover?
- Did Marshall paddle his limbs during the event?
- Did he lose control of his bladder?
- Did he lose control of his bowels?
- Did Mychael seem confused after the episode?
- Did Nick run into walls or otherwise appear to be blind after the incident?
- How long did this abnormal behavior persist?

This is time-consuming and the dialogue that results can feel very stiff and stilted. An assembly-line list of questions does not allow the client ample opportunity to expand upon his/her views.

For this reason, open-ended questions can be helpful because, unlike closed-ended questions, they are exploratory. They invite the client to share beyond a one-word or abbreviated answer.(33) In that respect, open-ended questions offer the client the floor to speak more freely.(33) This invitation helps to build the interpersonal relationship between the client and the veterinarian.(34)

Clients are likely to feel valued and respected as a partner in patient care. Clients that feel heard may be more likely to comply with recommendations. They also may be more likely to share questions or concerns because this questioning style opens up the opportunity for dialogue.

Clients are able to respond to open-ended questions with their own unique perspective.(33, 35) This allows them to share their thoughts, ideas, concerns, and emotions. (35) The words they use are their own. The descriptions that they provide are diverse and, without prompting, clients may share precisely what the veterinarian needed to ask.(36, 37)

Let us return to the case of syncope versus seizure. Rather than draw upon our list of closed-ended questions, use an open-ended one. Examples of appropriate open-ended questions for this case include:

- Tell me what you saw when Boo had this episode.
- Describe what you saw Beau do.
- Share with me what you observed.
- Paint me a picture of what it looked like to you.
- How would you describe what you saw?

Open-ended questions may insert *can you* or *please* to soften the request and make it seem more inviting. The same questions above could be transformed into:

- Can you please tell me what you saw when Boo had this episode?
- Please describe what you saw Beau do.
- Can you share with me what you observed?
- Can you paint me a picture of what it looked like to you?
- Can you please describe what you saw?

Client responses to open-ended questions are varied and diverse. Instead of being forced into pre-determined options for answers, clients are able to share their insight, on their own terms, in a way that is comfortable for them.

In addition, because open-ended questions allow clients to talk through their experiences, clients' memories may be jogged regarding important details surrounding the episode. Open-ended questions may also flush out areas of the case that the veterinarian may not have considered asking about but might be relevant to patient outcome or care.

It is advisable to consider the veterinary consultation as a funnel, in which both open-ended and closed-ended questions have their place.(33) Open-ended questions are a good starting point for the consultation because they provide clients with the opportunity to share what is on their minds.(33) Veterinarians may then clarify what has been shared or fill in the gaps by asking appropriate closed-ended questions as follow-up.(33)

4.4 Using Acronyms to Facilitate History-Taking

In addition to funneling the flow of conversation from open- to closed-ended questions, the clinician can use acronyms to recall which questions to ask. For example, in human medicine the acronym, SOCRATES, is typically referenced to elicit a thorough history for pain: (38–41)

- **S**ite of pain: Where is the pain located?
- **O**nset of pain: When did the pain start?
- **C**haracter of pain: How would you describe the pain?
- **R**adiation: Does the pain appear to migrate to other areas?
- **A**ssociation: Does the pain appear to be associated with any other factors?
- **T**ime course: Does the pain occur or recur at a certain time of day?
- **E**xacerbating: Does anything appear to make the pain worse?
- **S**everity: How would you rate the pain, from 1–10?

Although SOCRATES was developed to prompt medical doctors to ask follow-up questions related to the presenting complaint of pain, the acronym could be adapted for use in veterinary medicine. For example, let us return to the case of the limping dog. The client could provide responses to all but the question concerning the character of the pain. Without anthropomorphizing, it would be difficult for the client to describe the character of the pain as burning, throbbing, or a dull ache. However, the client could relay a significant amount of information about the other queries.

4.5 Client Expectations for the Patient

Client expectations should be determined through history-taking and incorporated into the "S" of the SOAP note. Although the majority of patients that are evaluated by veterinarians in small animal practice are intended to be companions, the purpose or the function of the patient should be established. It is important to know, for example, whether the client intends to breed the patient. If answered in the affirmative, this opens the door for conversation about the client's level of experience in the breeding circuit and invites discussion regarding breed predispositions to disease, behavioral considerations, and potential complications.

It is equally important to know if the patient is intended to be a therapy or working dog and, if so, what, if any, special requirements exist for medical management. For example, working police dogs that are relied upon for scent tracking tend not to receive intranasal vaccinations for fear that these may hinder their sense of smell.

If the patient is a horse, client expectations are equally important. Is this horse intended to be a "pasture pony" or a show horse? Certain medications are banned from use in the racetrack industry, so here again, a working knowledge of the horse's intended function is critical.

4.6 Lifestyle and History-Taking

Lifestyle refers to whether the patient is indoor, outdoor, or indoor/outdoor. For example, it is important to know whether a feline patient will experience outdoor living in order to assess its risk for contracting feline leukemia virus (FeLV) or feline immunodeficiency virus (FIV).

Lifestyle also includes pertinent information about the patient's home environment, specifically what and whom the patient encounters daily. Think about a stray cat that has recently been taken into a home. It is important for the veterinarian to establish with whom the cat will come into contact to minimize the risk that other pets in the household will contract communicable diseases. Alternatively, consider a cat that has just been diagnosed with toxoplasmosis. In this instance, it is critical that the veterinarian establish if there is a human pregnancy in the household to encourage dialogue about mitigating risk.

4.7 Activity Level

Another aspect of patient health that belongs in the "S" of the SOAP note is activity level. Activity level is important, particularly when meeting a new patient for the first time, because it provides a baseline against which subsequent behavior can be compared.

As an example, let us think about a patient that has been historically described as "hyperactive." If that same patient were to present months later for lethargy, the veterinarian's index of concern would be raised much more so than if a typically sedate patient presented for being "quiet."

Activity level is also important because it helps the veterinarian assess risk. Musculoskeletal injuries, for instance, are common in Frisbee-chasing dogs. Understanding which activities patients participate in can initiate conversations about patient safety and wellness *before* problems arise.

4.8 The Travel History and Serological Status

The "S" of the SOAP note should also make note of travel history and serological status in order to assess prior exposure to and current or future risk of acquiring infectious disease.

Think about heartworm infection in dogs. Although it has been diagnosed globally, heartworm (HW) infection is regionally endemic.(42) Furthermore, when patients and their human families travel from non-endemic to endemic regions, risk of acquiring the disease is elevated. When the now infected patient returns to the non-endemic region, a naïve population is potentially exposed to the disease.(43)

In clinical practice, it is advisable to know the serological status of cats with regards to FeLV and FIV. Feline patients are typically tested as kittens or at time of adoption via a single tabletop test, such as the SNAP FeLV/FIV Combo.

In canine practice, serological status is most typically reported for:

- HW
    - *Dirofilaria immitis*
- Lyme disease (L)
    - *Borrelia burgdorferi*
- *Ehrlichia* (E)
    - *Ehrlichia canis*
    - *Ehrlichia ewingii*
- *Anaplasma* (A)
    - *Anaplasma phagocytophilium*
    - *Anaplasma platys.*

Canine patients are typically evaluated for these six infectious diseases via a single tabletop test, such as the Snap 4Dx Plus. Because such tests are typically repeated in dogs annually, clients that are new to the practice may be able to provide past medical records with baseline serological data.

4.9 Diet History

A thorough diet history should be taken and included in the "S" of the SOAP note. The most pressing details include:

- What is the patient eating?
- What is the quantity of food that the patient consumes per day?
- Is the patient fed meals or ad libitum ("free fed")?
- If fed meals, how many meals per day?

It is also important to discuss the type of diet that is consumed. Knowing if the patient is fed a commercial or homemade, cooked or raw, meat-based or vegetarian diet is critical to the maintenance of patient health: (44–47)

- If the diet is a commercial brand, is it appropriate for the patient's life stage?
- If the diet is raw, is the client aware of the risks?
- If the diet is vegetarian and the patient is a cat, has taurine been supplemented so that the cat does not develop retinopathy or dilated cardiomyopathy (DCM)?

In order to be comprehensive, the diet history must also include all other treats, including table food.(44)

A 2008 study by Laflamme et al. demonstrates the abundance of snacks given to companion animals: in the United States and Australia, 56.8% of dogs and 26.1% of cats received treats daily.(48) These are contributing factors in the epidemic of weight gain.(49–53)

Increased body weight impairs wellness.(49) Overweight and obese dogs are predisposed to degenerative orthopedic diseases, such as osteoarthritis, as well as the development of insulin resistance, causing diabetes mellitus.(54–61)

Clinicians that do not expand the dietary history do their patients a disservice. They are missing key talking points and opportunity areas to engage in dialogue about fostering healthier eating habits.

For this reason, diet history must include anything the patient ingests, including vitamins, supplements, and snacks used to assist with medicating. Dietary supplements, including herbs, minerals, vitamins, and essential oils are increasingly popular in veterinary medicine as many products claim to prevent or manage disease.(48, 62–64)

Knowledge of supplements is critical because some may interact with medications if not spaced appropriately. For example, iron decreases absorption of doxycycline and therefore needs to be given several hours before or after a doxycycline dose.(65)

4.10 Past Pertinent Medical Care and History-Taking

The "S" in the SOAP note should also address the patient's past pertinent medical history with regards to preventative care, including, but not limited to:

- Patient identification
    - microchip
    - tattoo

- Vaccination status

  - current/up-to-date
  - overdue
  - unknown vaccination history
  - naïve/never vaccinated

- At-home dental care

  - dental treats or chews
  - dental rinses
  - water additives
  - tooth brushing

- Prior inpatient dental care

  - dental radiographs
  - dental prophylaxis
  - extractions

- Pharmaceutical prophylaxis

  - fleas
  - ticks
  - heartworms
  - gastrointestinal parasites.

If a client presents documentation of any of these, such documentation should be recorded for the benefit of future consultations.

Any other relevant familial, medical, anesthetic, surgical, or reproductive history belongs in the "S."

When patients present for a recheck appointment, their response to therapy should also be included in the "S" of the SOAP note.

4.11 Other Considerations for History-Taking

Other items that are documented in the "S" of the SOAP note include the clinician's subjective observations, such as descriptions of the patient's appearance following over-night hospitalization. For example, the veterinarian may write that the patient *looks brighter than yesterday.*(2)

The clinician may also choose to comment on the patient's behavioral responses:

- The patient hisses and spits at the front of the cat carrier
- The patient comes out of the cat carrier on its own if the door is opened during history-taking

- The patient attempts to bite if its feet are touched
- The patient is not tolerant of scruffing
- The patient tolerates gentle restraint, such as toweling
- The patient is reactive to direct eye contact
- The patient prefers to be examined on the floor rather than the exam room table.

In addition, the "S" of the SOAP note may incorporate the opinions of other consultants. For example, following a referral to a specialty service, the veterinarian may write that *the neurologist prioritizes a diagnosis of cancer.*

4.12 The Use of History Questionnaires

Keeping track of all the information that belongs in the "S" can be daunting.

- How can one possibly remember to ask every question, every time?
- How can a clinician be expected to stay on time, assuming that each client receives the same broad series of questions?

Some practices provide clients with questionnaires to augment the veterinarian's history-taking. These forms can be provided electronically to clients in advance of making the appointment, or these can be distributed and completed at the time of check-in.

Refer to Figures 4.1 and 4.2 for two examples of what these checklists may look like.

Veterinary team members' opinions about questionnaires vary widely. Some view them as a treasure chest of vital information. Others see them as a hindrance because they ask primarily closed-ended questions. Others take on a combined approach, using the questionnaire to obtain baseline data, then allowing the clinician the freedom to expand upon and clarify client responses.

4.13 Emotions Influence Subjective Data

Unlike objective data, subjective data may be influenced by past experiences and the emotions that are tied to them. History is a powerful reminder. It may trigger surprising reactions to the present when we least expect them.

Clients who react to benign news with strong emotions may have baggage from the past that they are bringing to the table. This is not something that the veterinary team may be aware of; however, when these situations arise, our gut reaction is to label the client as being overreactive.

Avoid this knee-jerk reaction whenever possible and instead, take care to elicit the client's perspective. It is important to understand where the client is coming from, so that we can address the client's concern head-on, whatever it may be. What may initially strike us as irrational may make perfect sense if we take the time to look beneath the surface.

HISTORY CHECKLIST

Please complete the following questions about your dog's health so that our team is able to assist you best

REASON(S) FOR TODAY'S VISIT
_____
_____
_____

WHAT IS YOUR GREATEST CONCERN?
_____
_____
_____

PATIENT DEMOGRAPHICS & IDENTIFICATION
- ❏ Age of patient: _____
- ❏ Breed of patient: _____
- ❏ Sex of patient: Male / Female
- ❏ Sexual status of patient: Spayed / Neutered / Not Sure
- ❏ If not neutered, do you plan to breed your dog? No / Yes
- ❏ Does your dog have a microchip? No/ Yes
- ❏ If yes: what is the identification number? _____

GENERAL
- ❏ How long have you owned your dog? _____
- ❏ Where did s/he come from? _____
- ❏ Is your dog a service or therapy dog? _____

LIFESTYLE
- ❏ Is your dog…? Indoor / Outdoor / Indoor-Outdoor
- ❏ Are there other pets at home? No / Yes: _____
- ❏ Do you ever board your dog? _____
- ❏ Do you take your dog to a groomer? _____
- ❏ Do you take your dog to doggie day care? _____
- ❏ Do you take your dog to the park? _____
- ❏ Do you travel with your dog? No / Yes: If yes, to what states/ countries: _____
- ❏ What kind of exercise does your dog do? _____

ENVIRONMENT
- ❏ Do you have any of the following person(s) in your home? Children; elderly; immune-compromised individuals, including those receiving chemotherapy? _____

BEHAVIOR
- ❏ Do you have any behavioral concerns about your dog? No / Yes: _____

Figure 4.1 Sample history questionnaire for a new client/dog-owner

NUTRITION	❑ What kind of dog food do you feed? How often?
	❑ What kinds of snacks do you give your dog?
	❑ Have you noticed unintentional changes in weight? No / Yes:
	❑ Have you noticed any vomiting or diarrhea? No / Yes:
PARASITE CONTROL	❑ Have you noticed any fleas or ticks on your dog? No / Yes
	❑ Please list any flea or tick control products your dog is currently receiving:
	❑ Do you protect your dog against fleas and ticks year-round? No / Yes
	❑ Has your dog been tested this year for heartworm disease? No/ Yes
	❑ If so, was s/he negative? No/ Yes
	❑ Please list any heartworm products your dog is currently receiving:
	❑ Do you protect your dog against heartworm disease year-round? No / Yes
VACCINATIONS	❑ Please note any vaccinations your dog has received
	❑ Do you have any concerns about vaccinations that your dog has received in the past or that your dog is due for today? No/Yes:
DENTAL CARE & PAST MEDICAL CARE	❑ Do you brush your dog's teeth? No/ Yes: ____ If so, how often?
	❑ Has your dog had any serious medical issues in the past? No/Yes:
	❑ Has your dog been diagnosed with any chronic diseases? No/Yes:
	❑ Does your dog receive any prescription medications? No/Yes:
	❑ Does your dog receive any over-the-counter medications? No/Yes:
	❑ Does your dog receive any vitamins or supplements? No/Yes:

Figure 4.1 continued

HISTORY CHECKLIST

Please complete the following questions about your cat's health so that our team is able to assist you best

REASON(S) FOR TODAY'S VISIT
_____
_____
_____

WHAT IS YOUR GREATEST CONCERN?
_____
_____
_____

PATIENT DEMOGRAPHICS & IDENTIFICATION
❏ Age of patient: _____
❏ Breed of patient: _____
❏ Sex of patient: Male / Female
❏ Sexual status of patient: Spayed / Neutered / Not Sure
❏ If not neutered, do you plan to breed your cat? No / Yes
❏ Does your cat have a microchip? No/ Yes
❏ If yes: what is the identification number? _____

GENERAL
❏ How long have you owned your cat? _____
❏ Where did s/he come from? _____
❏ Has your cat been tested for feline leukemia (FeLV)? No / Yes: ___
❏ Has your cat been tested for feline immunodeficiency virus (FIV)? No / Yes: _____

LIFESTYLE
❏ Is your cat…? Indoor / Outdoor / Indoor-Outdoor
❏ Are there other pets at home? No / Yes: _____
❏ Do you ever board your cat? _____
❏ Do you take your cat to a groomer? _____
❏ Do you travel with your cat? No / Yes: If yes, to what states/countries: _____

ENVIRONMENT
❏ Do you have any of the following person(s) in your home? Children; elderly; immune-compromised individuals, including those receiving chemotherapy? _____

BEHAVIOR
❏ Does your cat urinate or defecate outside of the litter box? No / Yes: _____
❏ Do you have any behavioral concerns about your cat? No / Yes: _____

Figure 4.2 Sample history questionnaire for a new client/cat-owner

NUTRITION	❏ What kind of cat food do you feed? How often?
	❏ What kinds of snacks do you give your cat?
	❏ Have you noticed unintentional changes in weight? No / Yes:
	❏ Have you noticed any vomiting or diarrhea? No / Yes:
PARASITE CONTROL	❏ Have you noticed any fleas or ticks on your cat? No / Yes
	❏ Please list any flea or tick control products your cat is currently receiving:
	❏ Do you protect your cat against fleas and ticks year-round? No / Yes
	❏ Please list any heartworm products your cat is currently receiving:
	❏ Do you protect your cat against heartworm disease year-round? No / Yes
VACCINATIONS	❏ Please note any vaccinations your cat has received
	❏ Do you have any concerns about vaccinations that your cat has received in the past or that your cat is due for today? No/Yes:
DENTAL CARE & PAST MEDICAL CARE	❏ Do you brush your cat's teeth? No/ Yes:
	If so, how often?
	❏ Has your cat had any serious medical issues in the past? No/Yes:
	❏ Has your cat been diagnosed with any chronic diseases? No/Yes:
	❏ Does your cat receive any prescription medications? No/Yes:
	❏ Does your cat receive any over-the-counter medications? No/Yes:
	❏ Does your cat receive any vitamins or supplements? No/Yes:

Figure 4.2 continued

Consider, for example, the client whose adult dog recently succumbed to lymphoma. That dog had first presented to a colleague with palpable lymphadenopathy under the jawline and in front of the shoulder blades. The client has since adopted a new puppy from the local animal shelter, which administered its first round of vaccinations. She is here today with the puppy for a wellness visit. This is her first time meeting you. You have no knowledge of her past history. During physical examination, you find a lump at the level of the right shoulder. You suspect it is secondary to vaccination and come across as blasé when describing it to the client. You are taken aback because the client starts to sob. You don't understand her reaction unless you know her back story, and that she automatically assumes the lump you found on her puppy is cancerous.

Eliciting the client's perspective is an essential part of history-taking. Eliciting the client's perspective refers to an active attempt by the veterinary team to explore the client's beliefs, concerns, or expectations.(33, 66, 67) Doing so encourages the client to share what is on his/her mind. It also helps to provide context for the client's reactions to circumstances or situations.

END-OF-CHAPTER SUMMARY

The "S" in SOAP notes stands for *subjective.*

In order to be complete, this *subjective* portion of the medical record should include:

- Patient signalment

  - age
  - sex
  - sexual status

    - male intact (MI) or entire male
    - male castrated (MC) or male neutered (MN)
    - female intact (FI) or entire female
    - female spayed (FS) or female neutered (FN)

  - breed and species

- Identifying features

  - coat color

- Presenting or chief complaint (cc)
- Client expectations
- Patient lifestyle
- Activity level

- Travel history
- Serological status
- Diet history
- Current medications, including over-the-counter vitamins and supplements
- Past pertinent health history, including familial, medical, surgical, and reproductive histories
- Vaccination status
- Current preventative care measures
- Past pertinent diagnostic tests and test results
- Past pertinent therapeutic trials and outcomes.

History-taking is the process by which this patient-specific data is gathered.

There are many different approaches to history-taking, including the five Ws and SOCRATES.

One of the most popular approaches is the use of the question funnel. History-taking begins with an open-ended question to invite the client to share his/her perspective. The clinician then follows up with closed-ended questions in order to clarify details or obtain specific key features that are relevant to patient health.

References

1. Cameron S, Turtle-song I. Learning to write case notes using the SOAP format. J Couns Dev. 2002;80(3):286–292.
2. Rockett J, Lattanzio C, Christensen C. The Veterinary Technician's Guide to Writing SOAPS: A Workbook for Critical Thinking. Heyburn, Idaho: Rockett House Publishing LLC; 2013.
3. Borcherding S. Documentation Manual for Writing SOAP Notes in Occupational Therapy. 2nd ed. Thorofare, NJ: SLACK Incorporated; 2005.
4. Kettenbach G. Writing Patient/Client Notes: Ensuring Accuracy in Documentation. 4th ed. Philadelphia: F.A. Davis Company; 2004. 248 pp.
5. Kettenbach G. Writing SOAP Notes: With Patient/Client Management Formats. 3rd ed. Philadelphia: F.A. Davis Company; 2004.
6. Rich EC, Crowson TW, Harris IB. The diagnostic value of the medical history. Perceptions of internal medicine physicians. Arch Intern Med. 1987;147(11):1957–1960.
7. Lichstein PR. The Medical Interview. In: Walker HK, Hall WD, Hurst JW, editors. Clinical Methods: The History, Physical, and Laboratory Examinations. Boston: Butterworths; 1990.
8. Bickley LS, Szilagyi PG, Bates B. Bates' Guide to Physical Examination and History-Taking. 11th ed. Philadelphia: Wolters Kluwer Health/Lippincott Williams & Wilkins; 2013. xxv, 994 pp.
9. Englar RE. Performing the Small Animal Physical Examination. Hoboken, NJ: Wiley; 2017.
10. Gough A, Thomas A. Breed Predispositions to Disease in Dogs and Cats. 2nd ed. Chichester, West Sussex; Ames, Iowa: Wiley-Blackwell; 2010. xvii, 330 pp.
11. Camacho P, Fan H, Liu Z, He JQ. Small mammalian animal models of heart disease. Am J Cardiovasc Dis. 2016;6(3):70–80.

12. Godiksen MT, Granstrom S, Koch J, Christiansen M. Hypertrophic cardiomyopathy in young Maine Coon cats caused by the p.A31P cMyBP-C mutation–the clinical significance of having the mutation. Acta Vet Scand. 2011;53:7.

13. Pedersen NC, Brucker L, Tessier NG, Liu H, Penedo MC, Hughes S, et al. The effect of genetic bottlenecks and inbreeding on the incidence of two major autoimmune diseases in standard poodles, sebaceous adenitis and Addison's disease. Canine Genet Epidemiol. 2015;2:14.

14. Klein SC, Peterson ME. Canine hypoadrenocorticism: part I. Can Vet J. 2010;51(1):63–69.

15. Famula TR, Belanger JM, Oberbauer AM. Heritability and complex segregation analysis of hypoadrenocorticism in the standard poodle. J Small Anim Pract. 2003;44(1):8–12.

16. Bishop MA, Steiner JM, Moore LE, Williams DA. Evaluation of the cationic trypsinogen gene for potential mutations in miniature schnauzers with pancreatitis. Can J Vet Res. 2004;68(4):315–318.

17. Bishop MA, Xenoulis PG, Levinski MD, Suchodolski JS, Steiner JM. Identification of variants of the SPINK1 gene and their association with pancreatitis in miniature schnauzers. Am J Vet Res. 2010;71(5):527–533.

18. Pinheiro D, Machado J, Viegas C, Baptista C, Bastos E, Magalhaes J, et al. Evaluation of biomarker canine-prostate specific arginine esterase (CPSE) for the diagnosis of benign prostatic hyperplasia. BMC Vet Res. 2017;13(1):76.

19. Barsanti JA, Finco DR. Canine prostatic diseases. Vet Clin North Am Small Anim Pract. 1986;16(3):587–599.

20. Journalistic Writing: Eastern Washington University; 2016. Available from: http://research.ewu.edu/c.php?g=403887

21. Arnold C, Cook T, Koyama D, Angeli E, Paiz JM. How to Write a Lead: Purdue University; 2013. Available from: https://owl.english.purdue.edu/owl/resource/735/05/

22. Dutton E, Dukes-McEwan J, Cripps PJ. Serum cardiac troponin I in canine syncope and seizures. J Vet Cardiol. 2017;19(1):1–13.

23. Grubb BP, Gerard G, Roush K, Temesy-Armos P, Elliott L, Hahn H, et al. Differentiation of convulsive syncope and epilepsy with head-up tilt testing. Ann Intern Med. 1991;115(11):871–876.

24. Linzer M, Grubb BP, Ho S, Ramakrishnan L, Bromfield E, Estes NA, 3rd. Cardiovascular causes of loss of consciousness in patients with presumed epilepsy: a cause of the increased sudden death rate in people with epilepsy? Am J Med. 1994;96(2):146–154.

25. Scheepers B, Clough P, Pickles C. The misdiagnosis of epilepsy: findings of a population study. Seizure. 1998;7(5):403–406.

26. Sheldon R, Rose S, Ritchie D, Connolly SJ, Koshman ML, Lee MA, et al. Historical criteria that distinguish syncope from seizures. J Am Coll Cardiol. 2002;40(1):142–148.

27. Smith D, Defalla BA, Chadwick DW. The misdiagnosis of epilepsy and the management of refractory epilepsy in a specialist clinic. QJM. 1999;92(1):15–23.

28. Zaidi A, Clough P, Cooper P, Scheepers B, Fitzpatrick AP. Misdiagnosis of epilepsy: many seizure-like attacks have a cardiovascular cause. J Am Coll Cardiol. 2000;36(1):181–184.

29. Chadwick D, Smith D. The misdiagnosis of epilepsy. BMJ. 2002;324(7336):495–496.

30. Werz MA. Idiopathic generalized tonic-clonic seizures limited to exercise in a young adult. Epilepsy Behav. 2005;6(1):98–101.

31. Schwartz DS, editor. The Syncopal Dog. World Small Animal Veterinary Association World Congress Proceedings; 2009; Sao Paulo, Brazil.

32. Thawley V, Silverstein D. Collapse. NAVC Clinician's Brief. 2012(November):14–15.

33. Hunter L, Shaw JR. What's in Your Communication Toolbox? Exceptional Veterinary Team. 2012(November/December):12–7.

34. Bard AM, Main DC, Haase AM, Whay HR, Roe EJ, Reyher KK. The future of veterinary communication: partnership or persuasion? A qualitative investigation of veterinary communication in the pursuit of client behaviour change. PLoS One. 2017;12(3):e0171380.

35. White PCL, Jennings NV, Renwick AR, Barker NHL. Questionnaires in ecology: a review of past use and recommendations for best practice. J Appl Ecol. 2005;42(3):421–430.

36. Reja U, Manfreda KL, Hlebec V, Vehovar V. Open-ended vs. close-ended questions in web questionnaires. Dev Appl Stat. 2003;19:158–177.

37. Huntley SJ, Mahlberg M, Wiegand V, van Gennip Y, Yang H, Dean RS, et al. Analysing the opinions of UK veterinarians on practice-based research using corpus linguistic and mathematical methods. Prev Vet Med. 2018;150:60–69.

38. Rae J. History Taking. London: OSCE Skills; 2017. Available from: http://www.osceskills.com/e-learning/subjects/patient-history-taking/

39. Clayton HA, Reschak GL, Gaynor SE, Creamer JL. A novel program to assess and manage pain. Medsurg Nurs. 2000;9(6):318–321, 317.

40. Briggs E. Assessment and expression of pain. Nurs Stand. 2010;25(2):35–38.

41. Reynoldson C, Stones C, Allsop M, Gardner P, Bennett MI, Closs SJ, et al. Assessing the quality and usability of smartphone apps for pain self-management. Pain Med. 2014;15(6):898–909.

42. Current Canine Guidelines for the Prevention, Diagnosis, and Management of Heartworm Infection in Dogs 2014. Available from: https://heartwormsociety.org/images/pdf/2014-AHS-Canine-Guidelines.pdf

43. Genchi C, Bowman D, Drake J. Canine heartworm disease (Dirofilaria immitis) in Western Europe: survey of veterinary awareness and perceptions. Parasit Vectors. 2014;7:206.

44. Baldwin K, Bartges J, Buffington T, Freeman LM, Grabow M, Legred J, et al. AAHA nutritional assessment guidelines for dogs and cats. J Am Anim Hosp Assoc. 2010;46(4):285–296.

45. Hayes KC. Nutritional problems in cats: taurine deficiency and vitamin A excess. Can Vet J. 1982;23(1):2–5.

46. Lenox C, Becvarova I, Archipow W. Metabolic bone disease and central retinal degeneration in a kitten due to nutritional inadequacy of an all-meat raw diet. JFMS Open Rep. 2015;1(1):2055116915579682.

47. Hayes KC, Trautwein EA. Taurine deficiency syndrome in cats. Vet Clin North Am Small Anim Pract. 1989;19(3):403–413.

48. Laflamme DP, Abood SK, Fascetti AJ, Fleeman LM, Freeman LM, Michel KE, et al. Pet feeding practices of dog and cat owners in the United States and Australia. J Am Vet Med Assoc. 2008;232(5):687–694.

49. Yam PS, Butowski CF, Chitty JL, Naughton G, Wiseman-Orr ML, Parkin T, et al. Impact of canine overweight and obesity on health-related quality of life. Prev Vet Med. 2016;127:64–69.

50. Sandoe P, Palmer C, Corr S, Astrup A, Bjornvad CR. Canine and feline obesity: a One Health perspective. Veterinary Record. 2014;175(24):610–616.

51. Day MJ. One Health: the small animal dimension. Veterinary Record. 2010;167(22):847–849.

52. Wynn SG, Witzel AL, Bartges JW, Moyers TS, Kirk CA. Prevalence of asymptomatic urinary tract infections in morbidly obese dogs. PeerJ. 2016;4:e1711.

53. Nijland ML, Stam F, Seidell JC. Overweight in dogs, but not in cats, is related to overweight in their owners. Public Health Nutrition. 2010;13(1):102–106.

54. White GA, Hobson-West P, Cobb K, Craigon J, Hammond R, Millar KM. Canine obesity: is there a difference between veterinarian and owner perception? J Small Anim Prac. 2011;52(12):622–626.

55. German AJ. The growing problem of obesity in dogs and cats. The Journal of Nutrition. 2006;136(7 Suppl):1940S-6S.

56. German AJ. Obesity in companion animals. Companion Animal Practice. 2010;32:42–50.

57. Lund EM, Armstrong PJ, Kirk CA, Klausner JS. Prevalence and risk factors for obesity in adult dogs from private U.S. veterinary practices. International Journal of Applied Research in Veterinary Medicine 2006;4:177–186.

58. Markwell PJ, Vanerk W, Parkin GD, Sloth CJ, Shantzchristienson T. Obesity in the dog. J Small Anim Prac. 1990;31(10):533–537.

59. Weeth LP, Fascetti AJ, Kass PH, Suter SE, Santos AM, Delaney SJ. Prevalence of obese dogs in a population of dogs with cancer. Am J Vet Res. 2007;68(4):389–398.

60. Kealy RD, Lawler DF, Ballam JM, Mantz SL, Biery DN, Greeley EH, et al. Effects of diet restriction on life span and age-related changes in dogs. J Am Vet Med Assoc. 2002;220:1315–1320.

61. Mattheeuws D, Rottiers R, Kaneko JJ, Vermeulen A. Diabetes mellitus in dogs: relationship of obesity to glucose tolerance and insulin response. Am J Vet Res. 1984;45(1):98–103.

62. Demirel G. Feeding practices for racehorses in Turkey. Journal Faculty Veterinary Medicine Istanbul University. 2006;32:79–86.

63. Burk AO, Williams CA. Feeding management practices and supplement use in top-level event horses. Comparative Exercise Physiology. 2008;5:85–93.

64. Ireland JL, Clegg PD, McGowan CM, McKane SA, Pinchbeck GL. A cross-sectional study of geriatric horses in the United Kingdom. Part 1: Demographics and management practices. Equine Vet J. 2011;43(1):30–36.

65. Plumb DC. Plumb's Veterinary Drug Handbook. 8th ed. Stockholm, Wisconsin Ames, Iowa: PharmaVet Inc.; 2015. 1279 pp.

66. Silverman J, Kurtz SM, Draper J. Skills for Communicating with Patients. 3rd ed. London; New York: Radcliffe Publishing; 2013. xviii, 305 pp.

67. Englar RE, Williams M, Weingand K. Applicability of the Calgary-Cambridge Guide to dog and cat owners for teaching veterinary clinical communications. J Vet Med Educ. 2016;43(2):143–169.

Chapter 5

The "O" in SOAP Notes

The "O" in SOAP notes stands for *objective*.(1–5) Objective data is inherently impartial and grounded in fact.(1–5) Objective data should not be influenced by emotion or opinion.(6)

An example of objective data is the patient's temperature: the patient is either febrile or not.

5.1 The Purpose of the "O" Section of SOAP Notes

The purpose of the "O" section of SOAP notes is to report patient-specific, measureable data. Accordingly, the following vital parameters are routinely recorded in this section:(2)

- Temperature (T)
    - recorded in °F or °C
- Pulse (P)
    - recorded in beats per minute (BPM)
- Respiratory rate (R)
    - recorded as breaths per minute
- Weight
    - kilograms (kg)
    - pounds (lb).

Vital signs should be documented at every visit to allow the veterinary team to establish what is considered *normal* for a given patient.

Not all patients fit the textbook's defined *reference range*. Some patients are outliers. That is, they consistently fall outside of the reference range as being either too low or too high. These deviations from the norm may be *normal* for that patient. The only way for us to learn what *normal* is for the patient is to routinely gather data and document it. This allows the veterinary team to identify trends and patterns.

For example, let us examine the case of a particularly hyperactive Labrador Retriever dog whose temperature has historically ranged from 103.0–103.5°F. Because this temperature is consistently documented in this patient's medical record as being mildly elevated, the veterinary team has an expectation of where this dog's temperature is likely to fall at the next visit.

If the patient's temperature is 103.2°F at the next visit and its physical examination is unremarkable, then its temperature is likely to be considered normal for this patient.

If, however, the patient's temperature now registers 105.7°F, then the veterinary team is more likely to suspect pathology and investigate further.

5.2 The Importance of Providing Units for Numerical Data

Units should be provided for numerical data. For example, weight should be recorded as pounds (lb), kilograms (kg), or both.

It is critical that the veterinarian be able to convert between units as needed using the appropriate conversion factors:

- To convert kilograms into pounds:

    - 1 kg = 2.2 lb
    - take the weight in kg and multiply by 2.2 lb/kg to obtain the weight in lb
    - Alternatively, take the weight in kg and divide by 0.45 kg/lb to obtain the weight in lb

- To convert pounds into kilograms:

    - 1 lb = 0.45 kg
    - take the weight in pounds and multiply by 0.45 kg/lb to obtain the weight in kg
    - alternatively, take the weight in pounds and divide by 2.2 lb/kg to obtain the weight in kg.

Most medication dosages are calculated based upon *milligrams (mg) per kg* of body weight.(7) However, some pharmaceuticals are calculated based upon body weight in *pounds*. For example:(7)

- Injectable cefovecin sodium (*Convenia*) is calculated at 3.6 mg/lb or 0.045 mL/lb, for antibiotic therapy
- Injectable maropitant citrate (*Cerenia*) is calculated at 0.45 mg/lb or 0.045 mL/lb, for acute vomiting.

Dosing errors are likely if the patient's body weight is assumed to be in pounds, but is actually written in kilograms, or vice versa.

The veterinary team may also make incorrect assumptions about weight gain or weight loss if units for weight are not included at all or if pounds and kilograms are inadvertently interchanged.

5.3 Other Numerical Values Often Recorded in the "O" Section of SOAP Notes

In addition to body weight, other numerical data has a place within "O."(2) For example:

- Baseline blood pressure (BP)
- Capillary refill time (CRT)
- Tabletop diagnostic test results, such as the SNAP FeLV/FIV Combo test
- Body condition score (BCS)

  - Nestlé-Purina 9-point scale

    – BCS 1/9 = emaciated
    – BCS 5/9 = ideal body weight
    – BCS 9/9 = obese

  - other scales may be used as long as the range is provided

    – BCS 3 is incorrect

      – does this mean BCS 3/9?
      – what is the scale?

    – BCS 3/5 is acceptable because it provides the reader with an understanding that 5 is the upper limit of the scaling system

      – BCS 3/5 is ideal
      – BCS 3/9 is underweight

- Muscle condition score (MCS) or muscle mass score (MMS)(8–10)

  - MCS of 3/3 equates to normal muscle mass. There is no muscle wasting
  - MCS of 2/3 equates to mild wasting of muscle mass
  - MCS of 1/3 equates to moderate wasting of muscle mass
  - MCS of 0/3 equates to severe wasting of muscle mass

- Diagnostic imaging findings

  - radiography
  - ultrasonography
  - echocardiography
  - fluoroscopy
  - computed tomography (CT) +/– contrast
  - magnetic resonance imaging (MRI) +/– contrast

- Blood, urinalysis and fecal test results
- Amount of subcutaneous fluids that were administered
- Amount of fluid tapped from the chest and/or abdominal cavity
- Amount of urine produced over "x" amount of time, as through a closed collection system.

Note that many of the above apply to inpatients only as opposed to new patients or outpatients.

When new patients present for a veterinary consultation, diagnostic tests are *not* typically included in the "O" section of SOAP notes because they take place at the end of the visit as part of the patient care plan.

For example, a veterinarian that is meeting a dog or cat for the first time may recommend a fecal flotation with microscopic examination for gastrointestinal parasites. However, the results will be reported in "P" rather than "O" to reflect that they are part of the patient care plan.

By contrast, a veterinarian tending to an inpatient that has its blood pressure rechecked every morning may opt to include today's BP reading in the "O" section of the SOAP note. In this case, taking a BP is considered to be part of the patient exam.

When documenting diagnostic test results in the medical record, it is important to be accurate. For example, it is inappropriate to document that the fecal analysis was "negative." The lack of observed ova is not a guarantee that the patient is free from parasitic infection.(11) It would be more medically accurate to notate that *no parasites or ova were observed.*

5.4 Documenting Physical Examination Findings in the "O" Section of SOAP Notes

In addition to numerical data, the "O" section of SOAP notes outlines physical examination findings.(1–5) Findings are typically reported in words; however, photographic additions to the medical record can be particularly useful in tracking the progression or resolution of dermatological or ophthalmological lesions.

To facilitate documentation of physical examination findings, some practices and teaching hospitals have designed stickers that outline the body by systems. Each is associated with a series of check-off boxes that allow the clinician to identify whether the system is normal or abnormal. Space is provided for clinicians to expand upon any abnormal finding. Refer to Figure 5.1 for an example.

The experienced clinician is likely to appreciate the efficiency that such a format provides. Clients may also appreciate that this format can be converted into a wellness "report card" that they can take home with them at the end of the consult.

This format is acceptable as long as all relevant findings have been documented.

However, the veterinary student or new graduate may not be ready for this abbreviated style of record-keeping. When a student checks the box marked "normal," is s/he

PHYSICAL EXAMINATION CHECKLIST FOR:

Patient Name _____

Patient ID# _____

DATE OF EXAM	_____
VITAL SIGNS	❏ Temperature: _____°F
	❏ Pulse: _____beats per minute
	❏ Respiratory Rate: _____breaths per minute
	❏ Weight: _____lb /// _____ kg
GENERAL APPEARANCE	❏ Normal
	❏ Abnormal:_____
INTEGUMENTARY	❏ Normal
	❏ Abnormal:_____
EYES/EARS/NOSE/ THROAT	❏ Normal
	❏ Abnormal:_____
CARDIOVASCULAR / RESPIRATORY	❏ Normal
	❏ Abnormal:_____
GASTROINTESTINAL	❏ Normal
	❏ Abnormal:_____
UROGENITAL	❏ Normal
	❏ Abnormal:_____
LYMPHATIC	❏ Normal
	❏ Abnormal:_____
MUSCULOSKELETAL	❏ Normal
	❏ Abnormal:_____
NERVOUS	❏ Normal
	❏ Abnormal:_____

Figure 5.1 Sample physical exam check-off sheet

truly aware of what *normal* means? What did s/he assess that gave the impression that the body was *normal*? Sometimes it is obvious, but more often it is not.

Consider, for example, the nervous system. If students are programmed to check the box marked, "normal," this implies that the following items were assessed on routine physical examination:

- Mentation
- Menace response
- Palpebral reflex
- Pupillary light reflex (PLR)

    - direct
    - consensual

- Conscious proprioceptive (CP) tests.

Were all of these items in fact assessed? Or was just one item assessed and that alone led the student to select the box marked "normal"?

Likewise, students have a tendency to select "normal" for the abdominal cavity. What does *normal* mean? Did they feel for the following organs?

- Stomach
- Spleen
- Liver
- Small intestine
- Large intestine

- Kidneys

    - left kidney
    - right kidney

- Urinary bladder.

If they felt for the organs listed above, which did they ultimately feel confident that they touched? Taking this a step further, which organs did they feel confident assessing size and shape or, in the case of the liver, margins?

A student's version of *normal* may be but a sliver of what *normal* means to an experienced clinician. Therefore, the author encourages students to get into the habit, at least initially, of writing out every examination in full, including the details surrounding normal findings. Over time, this builds confidence that each examination is complete and no system has been overlooked.

So how do veterinarians and veterinarians-in-training document physical examination findings?

There is no universal system of documentation.

Most clinicians develop a preferred approach as they journey through their formative years of veterinary college. This preference may be heavily influenced by the structure that was taught to them or required of them in their respective clinical rotations.

Many veterinarians start out with good habits that progressively decline with the pressures of clinical practice.

Remember that the medical record is a legal document. At the end of the day, it does not matter what you intended to document; it matters what made it into the written record.

There are several ways to approach documentation. Some clinicians write out their findings based upon the order in which they examined the patient – that is, from head to tail. Other veterinarians find it more helpful to break down the physical examination by systems.

Each veterinarian-in-training must 1) adopt his/her college's approach to record-keeping and 2) maintain good habits after graduation, even if that means adapting the school's approach to one that is better suited to meet the practice's needs.

It is beyond the scope of this text to describe every method of recording physical examination findings.

However, in my experience, I have found the following breakdown of systems to be effective:

- General appearance (GA)
- Integument (INTEG)
- Eyes/ears/nose/throat (EENT)
- Cardiovascular/respiratory (CV/RESP)
- Gastrointestinal (GI)
- Urogenital (URO)
- Lymphatic (LN)
- Musculoskeletal (MS)
- Nervous (NEURO).

Findings are reported for each category, including normals, until one's comfort level and consistency allow for *WNL*, within normal limits, or *NSF*, no significant findings.

For example, consider the "O" section of the SOAP note for a male canine patient that presents for a routine wellness examination:

- **General appearance (GA):** bright, alert, and responsive (BAR)
- **Integument (INTEG):** 1 × 2 mm alopecic scab – dorsolateral aspect of right pinna; 1 cm curvilinear superficial scratch along dorsal aspect of the bridge of the nose; otherwise WNL
- **Eyes/ears/nose/throat (EENT):** Dried brown crusting at medial canthi OU; scant ceruminous aural debris AU; no nasal discharge observed; non-painful on palpation over throat; no cough elicited when palpating the throat
- **Cardiovascular/respiratory (CV/RESP):** No murmur auscultated; sinus arrhythmia present; femoral pulses bilaterally symmetrical and strong; mucous membranes pink; normal bronchovesicular lung sounds
- **Gastrointestinal (GI):** soft, non-painful abdomen on palpation; negative for fluid wave; unable to feel stomach, liver, spleen; firm, formed feces palpable in descending colon; no palpable organomegaly; rectal examination WNL including normal size and shape of prostate and normal consistency to stool on rectal exam glove
- **Urogenital (URO):** Urinary bladder palpates as being moderate in size; non-reactive on urinary bladder palpation; unable to palpate either kidney
- **Lymphatic (LN):** Normal size, shape, texture, and symmetry – submandibular, pre-scapular, and popliteal; axillary and inguinal lymph nodes are not palpable
- **Musculoskeletal (MS):** normal gait and posture, no evidence of lameness
- **Nervous (NEURO):** Normal PLRs, palpebral reflex, and menace response; mentation normal.

Note that there is freedom to place physical examination findings in whichever category makes the most sense to the record-keeper. In the example above, pupillary light reflexes (PLRs) were included under the header, "Nervous (NEURO)"; however, they could also have fit within the header, "Eyes/ears/nose/throat (EENT)."

Note also that the level of detail, particularly for MS and NEURO, will vary depending upon the presenting complaint. For example, when describing the general wellness exam above, the findings under NEURO are typically restricted to mentation and cranial nerve tests. By contrast, an examination for an acutely recumbent Dachshund dog with presumptive intervertebral disk disease (IVDD) will be far more comprehensive. The veterinarian who is overseeing the Dachshund's care would be likely to address the following under NEURO: (12, 13)

- Gait
- Postural reactions
- Spinal reflexes
- Presence/absence of voluntary motor function in all four limbs
- Presence/absence of cervical pain
- Presence/absence of pain over the thoracic, lumbar, and sacral spine
- Presence/absence of conscious proprioceptive (CP) deficits as evidenced by knuckling in one or more limbs
- Presence/absence of deep pain
- Presence/absence of anal tone
- Normal/abnormal micturition
- Normal/abnormal defecation.

Because the nervous system is so complex, designed stickers or forms for the veterinarian to fill in can facilitate record-keeping. The same is true for the integumentary system, when working through a dermatological case, or the eye. Refer to Figures 5.2 through 5.4 for examples of each.

Note that my approach to the documentation of physical examination findings is not the only way. Some clinicians prefer to use the acronym, MENSCHRUG, as a reminder to assess every body system during a comprehensive physical examination.(6)

MENSCHRUG stands for: (6)

- **M**usculoskeletal
- **E**xternal
- **N**eurologic
- **S**ensory
- **C**ardiovascular
- **H**emolymphatic
- **R**espiratory
- **U**rogenital
- **G**astrointestinal.

It does not matter which method is used as long as the method is consistent, reproducible, and complete.

NEUROLOGICAL EXAMINATION CHECKLIST FOR:

Patient Name _____

Patient ID# _____

DATE OF EXAM	_____
MENTATION	❑ Normal ❑ Abnormal: _____
GAIT	❑ Normal ❑ Abnormal: _____

POSTURAL REACTIONS

❑ Knuckling:
_____LF _____RF _____LH _____RH

❑ Hopping:
_____LF _____RF _____LH _____RH

❑ Wheelbarrowing:
_____LF _____RF _____LH _____RH

❑ Placing (Tactile):
_____LF _____RF

❑ Placing (Visual):
_____LF _____RF

THORACIC LIMB REFLEXES

❑ Biceps Reflex
_____LF _____RF

❑ Triceps Reflex
_____LF _____RF

❑ Extensor Carpi Radialis Reflex
_____LF _____RF

❑ Withdrawal Reflex
_____LF _____ RF

PELVIC LIMB REFLEXES

❑ Patellar
_____LH _____RH

❑ Gastrocnemius Reflex
_____LH _____RH

❑ Cranial Tibial Muscle Reflex
_____LH _____RH

❑ Sciatic Nerve Reflex
_____LH _____RH

❑ Withdrawal Reflex
_____LH _____ RH

❑ Anal Reflex: _____

CRANIAL NERVES
- ❏ Pupil Symmetry: _____

- ❏ Pupillary Light Reflex (PLR):
    _____ OS (Direct)   _____OS (Consensual)
    _____OD (Direct)   _____OD (Consensual)

- ❏ Palpebral Reflex:
    _____OS   _____OD

- ❏ Menace Response
    _____OS   _____OD

- ❏ Strabismus: Y/N_____

- ❏ Nystagmus: Y/N_____

- ❏ CN V: Temporal/Masseter Muscle Symmetry
    _____

- ❏ CN IX/X: Swallowing
    _____

- ❏ CN XI: Trapezius Muscle
    _____

KEY
Reflexes
0 = absent
1 = depressed
2 = normal
3 = hyperactive

Postural Reactions
0 = paralysis
1 = some movement
2 = supports weight
3 = stumbles occasionally
4 = normal

Figure 5.2 Sample neurological exam check-off sheet

Take care to document all systems that were assessed during the physical examination and what findings were discovered.

In addition, write down what was not assessed and why. Recall from Chapter 1 that omissions weaken medical documentation. All healthcare industries, including veterinary medicine, are plagued by the phrase, "if it isn't charted, it didn't happen."(14–19)

INTEGUMENTARY EXAMINATION CHECKLIST FOR:

Patient Name _____

Patient ID# _____

DATE OF EXAM _____

LESIONS
Check all that apply and describe location(s)

❏ None
❏ Macules: _____
❏ Papules: _____
❏ Pustules: _____
❏ Vesicles: _____
❏ Crusts: _____
❏ Excoriations: _____
❏ Ulcers: _____
❏ Alopecia: _____
❏ Scales: _____
❏ Erythema: _____
❏ Pruritius: _____
❏ Wheals: _____
❏ Nodules: _____
❏ Tumors: _____
❏ Hyperpigmentation: _____
❏ Hyperkeratosis: _____

PARASITES

❏ None
❏ Fleas
❏ Ticks
❏ Lice
❏ Sarcoptes (based on microscopic exam)
❏ Demodex (based on microscopic exam)

DIAGNOSTIC TESTS

Mycology

❏ Woods Lamp
❏ KOH
❏ Culture

Skin Cytology

❏ Direct smear: _____
❏ Acetate tape impression: _____
❏ Superficial Skin Scraping: _____
❏ Deep Skin Scraping: _____

Ear Cytology

❏ AD: _____
❏ AS: _____

Biopsy

❏ _____

Figure 5.3 Sample dermatological exam check-off sheet

OPHTHALMIC EXAMINATION CHECKLIST FOR:

Patient Name _____

Patient ID# _____

DATE OF EXAM　　　　_____

LESIONS
Check all that apply and
describe location

❏ None
❏ Epiphora
　　　_____OS　　　_____OD

❏ Other ocular discharge
　　　_____OS　　　_____OD

❏ Blepharospasm
　　　_____OS　　　_____OD

❏ Blepharedema
　　　_____OS　　　_____OD

❏ Dystichiasis_____

❏ Trichiasis_____

❏ Conjunctivitis
　　　_____OS　　　_____OD

❏ Corneal Ulcer
　　　_____OS　　　_____OD

❏ Sclera: _____

❏ Iris: _____

❏ Lens:_____

❏ Fundic Exam: _____

❏ Other:_____

_____

_____

_____

_____

Figure 5.4　Sample ophthalmic exam check-off sheet

CRANIAL NERVES	❏ Pupil Symmetry: _____
	❏ Pupillary Light Reflex (PLR): _____OS (Direct) _____OS (Consensual) _____OD (Direct) _____OD (Consensual)
	❏ Palpebral Reflex: _____OS _____OD
	❏ Menace Response _____OS _____OD
	❏ Strabismus: Y/N_____
	❏ Nystagmus: Y/N_____
TESTS	❏ Retropulsion _____OS _____OD
	❏ Schirmer Tear Test (STT) _____OS _____OD
	❏ Fluorescein Staining _____OS _____OD
	❏ Tonometry _____OS _____OD

Figure 5.4 continued

5.5 Putting It All Together: The "S" and the "O"

Review Chapter 4 to consider the data that is typically included in the "S" section of SOAP notes and compare that data to what has been described here for the "O."

Note that at times, the separation between "S" and "O" is indistinct. You may question whether data belongs in "S" or "O," or in both. You may elect to include something in "S" whereas your colleague includes the same item in "O." You may find that I include something in "O" that you feel belongs in "S."

Examples of common areas of discrepancy include:

- Body condition score (BCS)
- Level of consciousness (LOC)
- Abnormal body odors, such as "acetone breath"(20, 21)
- Fur coat descriptions such as "dull" or "unkempt"
- Fecal consistency descriptions such as "soft" or "loose"
- Vomitus content descriptions such as "food" or "bile."

Depending upon one's perspective, any of these examples could justifiably belong in either "S" or "O."

At the end of the day, it is important not to stress over where data is housed. The SOAP note provides a foundation for a structured medical record. However, it does not dictate style or personal choice.(22) That is ultimately up to the individual clinician or practice.

The veterinarian is responsible for making certain that such data is included *somewhere* in the medical record. After all, the "S" and the "O" are simply a means to an end. They set the stage for the second half of the SOAP note, where data integration and critical thinking come into play.(23)

END-OF-CHAPTER SUMMARY

The "O" in SOAP notes stands for *objective.*

The purpose of this section is to report patient-specific, measurable data.

In order to be complete, this *objective* portion of the medical record should include:

- Vital parameters

    - temperature
    - pulse
    - respiratory rate
    - weight

- Other numerical data

    - body condition score (BCS)
    - muscle mass score (MMS) or muscle condition score (MCS)

- Physical examination findings.

Units should be provided for all numerical data, including certain vital parameters, such as weight. Most medication dosages are calculated based upon milligrams (mg) per kilogram (kg) of body weight. However, some pharmaceuticals are calculated based upon body weight in pounds (lb). Dosing errors are likely if units are assumed, rather than documented.

A breakdown of physical examination findings by system is most useful:

- General appearance (GA)
- Integument (INTEG)
- Eyes/ears/nose/throat (EENT)
- Cardiovascular/respiratory (CV/RESP)

- Gastrointestinal (GI)
- Urogenital (URO)
- Lymphatic (LN)
- Musculoskeletal (MS)
- Nervous (NEURO).

All findings are listed under each category, including those that are normal, until the veterinary student or new graduate is confident that s/he will not forget to examine routine body parts on every patient. At that point, the individual may transition to writing *no significant findings* (NSF) or *within normal limits* (WNL) for all normal findings and list only the abnormal ones.

References

1. Cameron S, Turtle-song I. Learning to write case notes using the SOAP format. J Couns Dev. 2002;80(3):286–292.
2. Rockett J, Lattanzio C, Christensen C. The Veterinary Technician's Guide to Writing SOAPS: A Workbook for Critical Thinking. Heyburn, Idaho: Rockett House Publishing LLC; 2013.
3. Borcherding S. Documentation Manual for Writing SOAP Notes in Occupational Therapy. 2nd ed. Thorofare, NJ: SLACK Incorporated; 2005.
4. Kettenbach G. Writing Patient/Client Notes: Ensuring Accuracy in Documentation. 4th ed. Philadelphia: F.A. Davis Company; 2004. 248 pp.
5. Kettenbach G. Writing SOAP Notes: With Patient/Client Management Formats. 3rd ed. Philadelphia: F.A. Davis Company; 2004.
6. Riegger MH. Using S.O.A.P. Is Good Medicine. DVM360; 2011.
7. Plumb DC. Plumb's Veterinary Drug Handbook. 8th ed. Stockholm, Wisconsin Ames, Iowa: PharmaVet Inc.; 2015. 1279 pp.
8. Chandler M. Nutrition for the Surgical Patient. In: Langley-Hobbs SJ, Demetriou JL, Ladlow JF, editors. Feline Soft Tissue and General Surgery. St. Louis: Saunders Elsevier; 2014. pp. 55–58.
9. Michel KE, Anderson W, Cupp C, Laflamme DP. Correlation of a feline muscle mass score with body composition determined by dual-energy X-ray absorptiometry. The British Journal of Nutrition. 2011;106 Suppl 1:S57-9.
10. Englar RE. Performing the Small Animal Physical Examination. Hoboken, NJ: Wiley; 2017.
11. Wigdor M. A study of the fecal examinations of 1000 imported dogs. J Am Vet Med Assoc. 1920;9.
12. De Lahunta A, Glass E, Kent M. Veterinary Neuroanatomy and Clinical Neurology. 4th ed. St. Louis, MO: Elsevier; 2015.
13. Dewey CW, Da Costa RC. Practical Guide to Canine and Feline Neurology. 3rd ed. Chichester, West Sussex; Hoboken: Wiley-Blackwell; 2016. xi, 672 pp.
14. Trossman S. The documentation dilemma: nurses poised to address paperwork burden. The American Nurse. 2001;33(5):1–18.
15. Page A, editor. Keeping Patients Safe: Transforming the Work Environment of Nurses. Institute of Medicine (US) Committee on the Work Environment for Nurses and Patient Safety. Washington, DC: National Academies Press; 2004. Available from: https://www.ncbi.nlm.nih.gov/books/NBK216190/
16. Nguyen AVT, Nguyen DA. Learning from Medical Errors: Legal Issues. Abingdon, United Kingdom: Radcliffe Publishing, Ltd.; 2005.
17. Andrews A, St Aubyn B. "If it's not written down; it didn't happen." Journal of Community Nursing. 2015;29(5):20–22.

18. Catalano J. Nursing Now! Today's Issues, Tomorrow's Trends. 7th ed. Philadelphia, PA: F.A. Davis Company; 2015.

19. David G, Vinkhuyzen E. Medical records' dynamic nature. If it isn't written down, it didn't happen. And if it is written down, it might not be what it seems. J AHIMA. 2013;84(11):32–35.

20. Shirasu M, Touhara K. The scent of disease: volatile organic compounds of the human body related to disease and disorder. J Biochem. 2011;150(3):257–266.

21. Qiao Y, Gao Z, Liu Y, Cheng Y, Yu M, Zhao L, et al. Breath ketone testing: a new biomarker for diagnosis and therapeutic monitoring of diabetic ketosis. Biomed Res Int. 2014;2014:869186. https://www.ncbi.nlm.nih.gov/pmc/articles/PMC4037575/pdf/BMRI2014-869186.pdf

22. Robey T. The art of writing patient record notes. Virtual Mentor. 2011;13(7):482–484.

23. Fleenor J. SOAP Notes: The Down and Dirty on Squeaky Clean Documentation. Denver, CO: shift 4 publishing, LLC; 2007.

Chapter 6

The "A" in SOAP Notes

The "A" in SOAP notes stands for *assessment* or *analysis*.(1–5) The assessment is the veterinarian's opportunity to consolidate the information in "S" and "O" into a workable problem list.

Recall from Chapter 3 that the problem list is a summation of patient-specific clinical signs, ailments, and abnormalities.

Remember also that the problem list is not static: it represents the patient's health at one moment in time. As problems resolve, persist, or intensify, the list evolves.

As each case unfolds, problems may be added, subtracted, or linked to one another. In this way, the problem list is a starting point that steers the veterinarian towards one or more diagnoses.

Let us consider the case of a 4-year-old, male castrated (MC), Siamese cat that presents for stranguria. The history and physical examination findings of this patient have been outlined below. We will use this information to create a problem list.

"S"

Presenting complaint: Owner (O) awoke to patient (P) going in and out of litter box 5–10×. P produced very little urine. P proceeded to squat on carpet next to litter box and dribbled scant amount of peach-colored urine. P vocalized sharply – different cry than usual. O left for work; returned 10 hours later. No urine clumps or feces in litter box. O found P laying on its side, with what appeared to be abdominal contractions.

Laterally recumbent on presentation.

General: Purchased from breeder as a kitten.

Lifestyle/environment: Indoor-only, single-cat household, lives only with owner. No changes in environment. Two litter boxes in house: one in basement and one on first floor. No travel history. Never groomed/boarded.

Behavior: Has never eliminated outside litter box.

Diet: Friskies adult canned cat food: ½ can BID; Friskies adult dry kibble ad lib; Drinks tablespoon of 2% milk once/week; occasionally eats rotisserie chicken, white meat only.

Parasite control: Not on flea/tick/heartworm preventative.

Vaccinations: Overdue on rabies and FVRCP by 2 years.

Serological status: Reportedly negative for FeLV and FIV (no past medical records provided).

Dental care: No at-home tooth brushing, has never had teeth professionally cleaned.

Past pertinent medical history: Upper respiratory infection at 4 months old; treated with amoxicillin; patient developed diarrhea – resolved once medication completed.

"O"

T: 102.0°F
P: 220 beats per minute (bpm)
R: 62 breaths per minute
Weight: 3.7 kg/8.14 lb

Body condition score (BCS): 4/9

Muscle condition score (MCS): MCS 3/3 – no muscle wasting.

General appearance (GA): quiet.

Integument (INTEG): Sluggish skin elasticity/some skin tenting, otherwise within normal limits (WNL).

Eyes/ears/nose/throat (EENT): Moderate ceruminous aural debris AU, otherwise no significant findings (NSF).

Cardiovascular/respiratory (CV/RESP): Grade 1/6 parasternal systolic murmur; light pink, tacky mucous membranes; tachycardic; tachypneic.

Gastrointestinal (GI): Inconsistent abdominal straining, uncomfortable on abdominal palpation.

Urogenital (URO): large, rock-hard urinary bladder; gritty debris at tip of purplish, pulsating penis.

> **Lymphatic (LN):** bilaterally symmetrical, palpable submandibular, prescapular, and popliteal lymph nodes – soft and supple; unable to appreciate axillary or inguinal lymph nodes.
>
> **Musculoskeletal (MS):** laterally recumbent.
>
> **Nervous (NEURO):** dull mentation, less responsive than would expect for cat in clinic, responds only on abdominal palpation with lifting of head and guttural cry.

From the history and physical examination findings above, we can construct the following problem list:

1. Stranguria
2. Peach-colored urine
3. Minimal urine production
4. Abdominal contractions
5. Hard, enlarged urinary bladder
6. Penile discoloration
7. Penile pulsation
8. Blood clot at tip of penis
9. Vocalization
10. Progressive lethargy
11. Lateral recumbency
12. Dehydration, estimated 5–7%
13. Tachycardic
14. Grade 1/6 parasternal murmur
15. Tachypneic
16. Dull mentation
17. Responsive only on abdominal palpation.

Note that the order in which problems are listed may vary between clinicians.

Some clinicians list problems chronologically, based upon the order in which they present themselves in the history and physical exam. This strategy can be appreciated from the example above.

Other clinicians lump problems together so that like categories are near one another. Using this strategy, all problems linked to the urinary system would be listed near one another like so:

- Stranguria
- Peach-colored urine
- Minimal urine production
- Hard, enlarged urinary bladder
- Penile discoloration
- Penile pulsation
- Blood clot at penile tip.

Other clinicians prioritize the problem list in order of most to least importance, to prioritize patient care.

As with most other areas of medical documentation, there is no one *right* approach. With practice, you will establish which method comes most naturally to you.

As a student, I found it easier to start with a chronological approach so that I did not inadvertently leave any problems off the list.

As an experienced practicing clinician, I found it more helpful to prioritize problems based upon their severity. My plan of attack for patient care naturally followed the same order. Most important problems were addressed immediately. Least important problems could be tabled until the most pressing concern had been addressed or the patient was stable.

Let us review a second example of a 2-year-old, male intact (MI), Rottweiler dog that presents on emergency for acute vomiting.

"S"

Presenting complaint: Owner (O) awoke to three piles of vomit on carpet next to bed. Vomitus appeared to be undigested food. Stained carpet yellow. Two dogs in house. O unsure which dog vomited. Attitude of both dogs seemed normal so O fed them breakfast. Both dogs ate. Ten minutes after patient (P) ate, P started lip-smacking and hypersalivating. P vomited meal shortly after eating. O described active process with abdominal contractions. P drank water half-hour later. P proceeded to vomit within ten minutes of drinking water. Vomitus contained water and food. P has continued to dry heave intermittently for the past few hours. O hasn't seen patient defecate in two days.

General: Purchased from online advertisement, roughly six months ago

Lifestyle/environment: Primarily outdoor. Has free access to the garage. O noticed leak in the antifreeze container in the garage upon arrival home from work. Did not observe P consuming antifreeze. P comes in the house only at bedtime. Lives with one other large-breed canine mix (~65 lb). Reportedly, the two dogs get along. The other dog is not (as of now) symptomatic. P goes swimming 2–4×/month at local pond. Was at pond last week. Recently bathed at community dog wash event.

Behavior: Reportedly chases cats.

Nutrition: One can of Alpo BID; Old Roy dry kibble "large bowl" (unmeasured) BID; frequent table-scraps. Last night got into trash. May have ingested grease +/– tinfoil from baking turkey in oven.

Parasite control: Currently on topical, monthly, year-round flea preventative; currently taking seasonal oral heartworm preventative – both brands unknown.

Vaccinations: Overdue on rabies vaccination; has never received DA2PP (Distemper/Parvo) series to owner's knowledge

Serological status: Reportedly heartworm negative.

Dental care: No at-home tooth brushing, has never had teeth professionally cleaned. O feeds P rawhides to "reduce plaque."

Past pertinent medical history: Unknown prior to adoption six months ago.

"O"

T: 103.7°F
P: 98 beats per minute (bpm)
R: 36 breaths per minute
Weight: 61.4 kg/135 lb

BCS: 7/9

Muscle condition score (MCS): MCS 3/3 – no muscle wasting.

General appearance (GA): quiet, dull.

Integument (INTEG): Sluggish skin elasticity/some skin tenting, otherwise WNL.

Eyes/ears/nose/throat (EENT): NSF.

Cardiovascular/respiratory (CV/RESP): WNL – no murmurs/arrhythmias.

Gastrointestinal (GI): Increased GI sounds on auscultation. Small bowel palpates as having appreciably fluid contents. Mild crunching on abdominal palpation. "Prayer posture"/"play bow" stance is observed when abdominal palpation is discontinued – forelimbs are lower than hind limbs; unable to feel stomach/liver/spleen/descending colon.

Urogenital (URO): unable to palpate either kidney; small urinary bladder.

Lymphatic (LN): bilaterally symmetrical, palpable submandibular, prescapular, and popliteal lymph nodes; unable to appreciate axillary or inguinal lymph nodes.

Musculoskeletal (MS): limited motion/activity.

Nervous (NEURO): depressed mentation.

The history and physical examination findings of this patient have been outlined below. We will use this information to create a problem list.

1. No knowledge or record of receiving DA2PP vaccinations
2. Overdue on rabies vaccination
3. Acute vomiting
4. Febrile
5. Lip-licking
6. Hypersalivating
7. Swam in pond last week
8. Bathed at local dog wash recently
9. Got into trash/may have gotten into grease +/- tinfoil
10. Had access to leak in antifreeze container
11. Quiet
12. Depressed mentation
13. Dehydration, estimated 5–7%
14. "Prayer posture"/"Play bow" stance
15. Fluidy contents – small bowel
16. Lethargic
17. Cat-chaser.

Note that all problems are listed, even those that do not appear to be related to the primary problem. For example, the fact that this patient is historically interested in chasing cats is not relevant to the presenting complaint; however, to be thorough and to prevent cat chasing from being lost to follow-up, it needs to be included in the problem list.

Once the initial problem list has been developed from the "S" and the "O," each component is considered in light of what type of pathology could have caused or contributed to it. These potential explanations for each problem form a patient-specific list of differential diagnoses.

Lists of differential diagnoses should be thorough, but realistic. That is, for a differential diagnosis to be considered, it must be possible for that particular patient.

For example, it would be unreasonable to include as a differential diagnosis an infectious disease that does not even exist on the continent where a non-travelling, homebound patient resides.

On the other hand, it would be reasonable to include valley fever as a differential diagnosis for a patient that has travelled through or lived in the state of Arizona.

In addition to being relevant to the patient in question, differential diagnoses should be ranked in order of most to least likely. Clients are going to ask why disease "x" is more likely than disease "y." The veterinary team must be able to explain why patient-specific differentials are more or less probable in order to justify the proposed diagnostic work-up.(1–5)

Just as the problem list should not suffer from tunnel vision, the same holds true for the differential list. It may be tempting to zero in on one differential based upon pattern recognition. However, doing so can be dangerous for the patient by virtue of excluding other equally probable causes.

To facilitate keeping an open mind, several acronyms have been developed to guide clinicians through broad categories of causes that should be considered when compiling a list of differentials.

One such acronym is ***NITSCOMP DH***: (6)

- **N**eoplasia
- **I**nfectious
- **T**oxicities
- **S**tructural
- **C**ongenital

- **O**ther
- **M**etabolic
- **P**arasitic
- **D**iet
- **H**usbandry.

Let's revisit the case of the 2-year-old, unvaccinated, MI Rottweiler dog, and use the NITSCOMP DH acronym to flush out differential diagnoses for the problem list.

The current problem list for this patient has 17 entries. Each entry or problem requires its own differential list, although there is likely to be some degree of overlap. For example, both lip-licking and hypersalivating are suggestive of nausea. In other words, they overlap.

Areas of overlap are helpful because they consolidate the problem list. They may also suggest a common denominator for a given presentation. When a differential diagnosis is listed for more than one problem, the index of suspicion is raised: this one differential diagnosis could be correct.

Returning to the case of the vomiting dog, the acronym, NITSCOMP DH, helps us to consider the various differentials for the primary problem, vomiting:

- **N**eoplasia
    - gastrointestinal lymphoma

- **I**nfectious
    - parvovirus
    - bacterial gastroenteritis, such as leptospirosis

- **T**oxicities
    - ethylene glycol ingestion

- **S**tructural
    - intussusception
    - pyloric stenosis

- **C**ongenital
    - hiatal hernia

- **O**ther
  - foreign body
  - dysautonomia

- **M**etabolic
  - hypoadrenocorticism
  - pancreatitis
  - hepatitis
  - gastritis
  - non-infectious gastroenteritis

- **P**arasitic
  - roundworms
  - whipworms
  - hookworms
  - tapeworms
  - *Giardia*

- **D**iet
  - dietary indiscretion
  - food sensitivity
  - food allergy

- **H**usbandry
  - see diet.

Note that not every possible cause of vomiting is listed above. This is because the goal of the acronym is not to be exhaustive. The goal is to promote critical thinking and data integration that encourages the veterinarian to consider that which is most likely. Causes that are listed are considered more likely than those that are not.

When a veterinary student is creating lists of differential diagnoses for the first time, it is prudent to include more items than less. Items that are included on the list are considered possible until they are ruled out.

If an item never makes it onto the list in the first place, it is unlikely to be considered and could result in a missed opportunity for diagnosis.

NITSCOMP DH is not the only acronym in existence. Many veterinarians are more familiar with an alternate approach, the DAMNIT scheme. Depending upon how many letters of each (D, A, M, N, I, and T) are incorporated into the acronym, there are several versions, one of which is outlined below: (7, 8)

- **D**egenerative
- **D**evelopmental
- **A**nomalous
- **A**utoimmune
- **M**etabolic
- **M**ental

- **N**utritional
- **N**eoplastic
- **I**nflammatory
- **I**nfectious
- **I**schemic

- **I**atrogenic
- **I**diopathic
- **T**raumatic
- **T**oxicity.

Some clinicians forego acronyms altogether and simply list out differential diagnoses. Returning to the example of the vomiting Rottweiler dog, this simplified approach to list-making may look something like this for the primary problem:

- Primary gastrointestinal (GI) disease

  - parvovirus
  - other infectious disease
  - foreign body
  - dietary indiscretion
  - food sensitivity
  - food allergy
  - GI parasites

- Secondary metabolic disease

  - hypoadrenocorticism
  - pancreatitis
  - hepatitis
  - acute renal failure
  - ethylene glycol ingestion
  - other toxin.

Three approaches to the same case have been presented here. Note that any of these three are acceptable tools that organize the "A" section of the SOAP note. All three fulfill their primary purpose: to summarize patient data in order to guide decision-making that leads to an appropriate case management plan for the patient.

END-OF-CHAPTER SUMMARY

The "A" in SOAP notes stands for *assessment* or *analysis.*

The purpose of this section is to consolidate the information that was obtained in "S" and "O" into a workable problem list.

In healthcare, problems refer to patient-specific clinical signs or abnormalities, including those that are identified through physical examination or laboratory results.

A problem list is therefore a summary of patient-specific issues.

A problem list is dynamic: it evolves alongside of patient care.

Problems may resolve, persist, or intensify.

Every problem on the problem list has one or more causes. The burden falls upon the clinician to identify these causes.

Sometimes, what has caused each problem is obvious. For example, a dog that ingests anticoagulant rodenticide presents with coagulopathies.

However, more often than not, the clinician must explore various possibilities for what may have caused each problem on the problem list. These possibilities are called differential diagnoses.

Differential diagnoses are listed by problem.

Patients with multiple problems will have multiple lists of differential diagnoses. Sometimes these lists overlap, pointing the clinician in the right direction of the most likely diagnosis.

Lists of differential diagnoses should be thorough, but realistic. In order to make the list, differential diagnoses should be possible for the patient in question. For example, pyometra is not an acceptable differential diagnosis for a male dog with polyuria/polydipsia unless the patient in question is a hermaphrodite.

Two acronyms may facilitate brainstorming sessions to develop lists of differential diagnoses: NITSCOMP DH and the DAMNIT scheme.

References

1. Cameron S, Turtle-song I. Learning to write case notes using the SOAP format. J Couns Dev. 2002;80(3):286–292.
2. Rockett J, Lattanzio C, Christensen C. The Veterinary Technician's Guide to Writing SOAPS: A Workbook for Critical Thinking. Heyburn, Idaho: Rockett House Publishing LLC; 2013.
3. Borcherding S. Documentation Manual for Writing SOAP Notes in Occupational Therapy. 2nd ed. Thorofare, NJ: SLACK Incorporated; 2005.
4. Kettenbach G. Writing Patient/Client Notes: Ensuring Accuracy in Documentation. 4th ed. Philadelphia: F.A. Davis Company; 2004. 248 pp.
5. Kettenbach G. Writing SOAP Notes: With Patient/Client Management Formats. 3rd ed. Philadelphia: F.A. Davis Company; 2004.
6. Riegger MH. Using S.O.A.P. Is Good Medicine. DVM360; 2011. Available from: http://veterinarynews.dvm360.com/using-soap-good-medicine.
7. Osborne CA. 'DAMN-IT' acronym offers practical diagnostic aid. DVM360 [Internet]; 2005. Available from: http://veterinarynews.dvm360.com/damn-it-acronym-offers-practical-diagnostic-aid
8. Lorenz MD, Neer TM, Demars PL. Small Animal Medical Diagnosis. 3rd ed. Ames, Iowa: Wiley-Blackwell; 2009. xv, 502 pp.

Chapter 7

The "P" in SOAP Notes

The "P" in SOAP notes stands for *plan.*(1–5) The plan outlines the veterinarian's intentions: what does s/he want to do, why, and in what timeframe, to address, medically manage, and (ideally) resolve the patient's problem(s).

The plan requires the veterinarian to consider that which is essential to patient care: what steps need to be taken now and which steps (if any) can be taken later?

A common approach in academia and private practice is to trisect the plan into: (6)

- Diagnostic recommendations
- Therapeutic recommendations
- Management recommendations or client communication notes.

Each category in this triad may be listed separately under "P" or all three categories may be lumped together. Either approach is considered appropriate as long as the clinician considers all three when formulating the master plan.

As a veterinary student, I felt most comfortable considering each category for "P" as a separate entity. This trend lasted until I felt comfortable that I would remember to consider all aspects of the patient care plan.

As my experience level grew in clinical practice, I felt it easier and more efficient to combine all three into a single "P."

7.1 Diagnostic Recommendations

Diagnostic recommendations suggest which patient tests to pursue and why.(6) The following are examples of diagnostic tests:

- Baseline bloodwork
    - complete blood count (CBC)
    - serum biochemistry profile
- "Stim tests," such as the ACTH stimulation test to diagnose adrenal insufficiency

- Urinalysis

  - urine specific gravity
  - urine dipstick
  - urine sediment cytology

- Fecal analysis

  - wet mounts
  - fecal flotation
  - Baermann technique

- Cytology

  - aural
  - blood smears
  - bone marrow aspirates
  - conjunctival
  - fine needle aspirates (FNAs)
  - tracheal wash

- Histology

  - excisional biopsies
  - incisional biopsies

- Imaging studies

  - radiography
  - ultrasonography
  - echocardiography
  - fluoroscopy
  - computed tomography (CT) +/– contrast
  - magnetic resonance imaging (MRI) +/– contrast

- Scoping

  - bronchoscopy
  - colonoscopy
  - endoscopy
  - guttural pouch examination (equine)
  - otoscopy
  - rhinoscopy

- Exploratory surgery
- Necropsy.

Many diagnostic recommendations, but not necessarily all, can be pursued in-house. Others may require sample submission to an outside diagnostic laboratory or referral of the patient.

Note that diagnostic recommendations vary in terms of turnaround time. Turnaround time is the time it takes for laboratory results to become available after the sample has been received by the diagnostic laboratory.

Turnaround time may be insignificant. For example, most tabletop ELISA snap test kits take ten minutes or less to register results.

However, turnaround time may be substantial. For example, a polymerase chain reaction (PCR) test for systemic mycoses typically takes up to three business days.(7)

It is important that turnaround time for results be shared with the client in advance of sample submission so that both clinician and client are on the same page in terms of expectations.

In cases where turnaround time for diagnostic test results is substantial, the clinician and client will need to come to an understanding as to how to proceed with patient care while waiting.

It is important to recognize that in these cases, particularly if the patient is symptomatic, diagnostic recommendations are not appropriate as the sole means of case management.

Recall the 4-year-old, castrated male Siamese cat that was introduced in Chapter 6. Let us return to this case to consider our diagnostic plan. Based upon pattern recognition and what information was shared in Chapter 6 concerning the history and physical examination findings, this cat is likely to have a urinary tract obstruction (UTO).

An appropriate diagnostic plan for this patient might include:

- CBC
- Serum biochemistry panel
- Urinalysis
- Urine culture
- Two-view abdominal radiographs to evaluate the urinary tract for evidence of stones
- Urethral plug analysis
- Electrocardiogram (ECG) to assess for arrhythmias

  - hyperkalemia-induced bradycardia is common in cats with UTO

- Echocardiogram if murmur persists and/or worsens.

Recall the second case that was introduced in Chapter 6: the 2-year-old, intact male (MI), Rottweiler dog that presented on emergency for acute vomiting. Based upon pattern recognition and what information was shared concerning the history and physical examination findings, this dog is likely to have succumbed to one or more of the following differentials:

- Infectious disease, such as parvovirus or leptospirosis
- Ethylene glycol toxicosis
- Foreign body ingestion (tinfoil)
- Gastrointestinal parasitism
- Gastrointestinal upset or pancreatitis secondary to dietary indiscretion.

An appropriate diagnostic plan for this patient might include:

- CBC
- Serum biochemistry panel
- Urine collection
- Urinalysis
- Fecal analysis
- Parvovirus ELISA snap test
- *Giardia* ELISA snap test
- cPL ELISA snap test
- Submission of blood and/or urine for real-time PCR test for leptospirosis.

7.2 Therapeutic Recommendations

Therapeutic recommendations are a second arm of case management aimed at addressing the patient's presenting complaint(s) and problem list.(6) The goal of therapeutic recommendations is to target clinical signs and provide some degree of relief, if not a cure.

The following are examples of therapeutic recommendations:

- Suggesting over-the-counter (OTC) medications or supplements
- Prescribing medications in-house or providing a script so that prescriptions can be filled elsewhere
- Providing supportive care

  - active warming
  - fluid therapy
  - nutritional support

- Admitting to the hospital for observation and professionally managed care
- Transitioning to at-home care
- Enrolling in a weight-loss program
- Implementing physical therapy.

Let us re-examine the case of the 4-year-old, castrated male, Siamese cat. An appropriate therapeutic plan for this cat might include:

- IV catheter placement
- IV fluid therapy: _[insert fluid type]_ at _[insert number]_mL/h for _[insert number]__ hours
- Recheck vital signs every _[insert number]_ hours
- Alert veterinarian if heart rate exceeds _[insert number]_ beats per minute or drops below _[insert number]_ bpm

- Alert veterinarian if respiratory rate exceeds _[insert number]_ breaths per minute or drops below _[insert number]_ breaths per minute
- Alert veterinarian if temperature exceeds _[insert number]_°F or drops below _[insert number]_°F
- Sedation of the patient with: _[insert drug name and concentration]_ at _[insert number]_mg, administered __[insert route]___ at _[insert time of administration]_
- Analgesia: _[insert drug name and concentration]_ at _[insert number]_mg, administered __[insert route]___ at _[insert time of administration]_
- Unblock patient with __[insert name and size of]__ urinary catheter
- Place __[insert name and size of]__ indwelling urinary catheter
- Set-up urine closed collection kit
- Place Elizabethan collar
- Reverse sedation with: _[insert drug name and concentration]_ at _[insert number]_ mg, administered __[insert route]___ at _[insert time of administration]_
- Maintain analgesia with _[insert drug name and concentration]_ at _[insert number]_mg, administered __[insert route]___ at _[insert time of administration]_. Repeat every __[insert number]___ hours as needed (PRN)
- Measure urine produced in closed collection kit every __[insert number]___ hours
- Offer water
- Offer ___[insert food name and type]____ beginning ___[insert time frame]_____.

7.3 Management Recommendations or Client Communication Notes

Appreciate how both diagnostic and therapeutic recommendations play an instrumental role in case management; however, neither will be effective without client communication. Client communication represents the third component of the "P" section of the SOAP note and serves as a written record of information that is shared with the client.

In this way, client communication notes protect the veterinarian against liability by serving as a legal report of the conversations that took place, including what the client consented to or, alternatively, if the client withheld consent.

To be complete, client communication notes should include information that is shared with the client about the patient's: (6)

- Presenting complaint
- Differential diagnoses
- Diagnostic recommendations
- Therapeutic recommendations
- Final diagnosis
- Prognosis.

To see how this looks on paper, let us recall the case of the 2-year-old, MI, Rottweiler dog that presented on emergency for acute vomiting.

Client communication notes for this patient could state that three options were discussed concerning the patient's vomiting.

Plan A includes a full diagnostic work-up:

* CBC
* Serum chemistry panel
* Urinalysis
* Two-view abdominal radiographs
* Parvovirus ELISA snap test
* *Giardia* ELISA snap test
* Real-time PCR of blood and/or urine to test for leptospirosis
* Hospitalization for intravenous fluid therapy.

Plan B includes a limited work-up:

* Parvovirus ELISA snap test

    * if positive, then hospitalize to treat for parvovirus
    * if negative, then hospitalize for observation, intravenous fluid therapy, and supportive care.

Plan C includes a bare-bones work-up:

* Subcutaneous fluid therapy
* Transition to outpatient care
* At-home anti-emetic therapy
* Nothing per os (NPO) for six hours with gradual reintroduction of water, followed by introduction of a bland diet.

Note that all plans provide pertinent details regarding the proposed type of care (inpatient vs. outpatient) and treatments (intravenous vs. subcutaneous fluid therapy).

However, as written above, these client communication notes are incomplete. Notes are incomplete because:

* It is unclear which plan the veterinarian is recommending
* There is no discussion about pros/cons of each option
* Plans A and B lack detail about the estimated length of stay in the hospital
* Plan A lacks detail on when the diagnostic test results are expected to be finalized
* Plan B lacks detail on when and how the patient will be reassessed
* Plan C lacks detail about when the client is expected to follow up and when the client should become concerned that Plan C is not working.

Details are the glue that holds the medical record together. When details are missing, the medical record loses value, particularly as a legal document.

Taking care to document details may seem inefficient. However, a detail-oriented approach is beneficial because it minimizes the opportunity for miscommunication.

It also reduces ambiguity that may lead to medical mistakes and other errors in decision-making.

In addition, a detail-oriented approach facilitates relationship-centered care. It ensures that the veterinarian and the client are on the same page in terms of patient care and expectations for patient outcomes.

Keep in mind that plans, like problem lists, are dynamic and are therefore expected to change as the needs for the patient change.

7.4 Putting It All Together: The "A" and the "P"

Just as the "S" and the "O" are philosophically linked, so, too, are the "A" and the "P." The "A" tells a story about what you, the veterinarian, think is going on. The "P" completes the story by sharing what you plan on doing about it.

Anyone can be trained to transcribe the "S" and the "O." However, it takes a true diagnostician to work through the "A" and the "P." Both require critical thinking and willingness to invest the time and energy to problem-solve.

Historically, the "A" and "P" are written top-to-bottom, meaning that the "A" appears first in the medical record, followed by the "P." Corresponding numbers are then assigned to the plan(s) that match(es) each problem.

For example, reconsider the case of the Rottweiler dog. Recall that the very first problem for this patient that was listed under "A" in Chapter 6 was:

1. No record of receiving DA2PP vaccinations.

Under "P," under the subcategory "diagnostic plan," any recommendation that addresses or clarifies the problem would also be labeled with a "1." For this specific case, the following aspect of the diagnostic plan would be listed:

1. Parvovirus ELISA snap test.

Note that not every problem in "A" may have a corresponding plan in "P." For example, the problem of "cat chasing" for the same patient may not have anything listed under "P" because the client already has established a way to manage this problem: the household does not include cats.

Note also that one action item under "P" may cover several problems listed in "A." In other words, the list under "P" does not have to be equal in size to the list under "A." In fact, it may be significantly shorter. For example, the action item of unblocking the 2-year-old, castrated male Siamese cat will address the following problems that had been outlined under "A":

*   Minimal urine production
*   Abdominal contractions

- Rock hard, large urinary bladder
- Penile discoloration
- Penile pulsation
- Blood clot at penile tip.

Not every clinician shares the same thought process. Accordingly, not every clinician prefers the top-to-bottom approach for placing the "A" and the "P" in the medical record. Some may prefer to place the "A" and "P" side by side to reinforce the links between the "A" and the "P." In the case of the Rottweiler, that would look something like this, for the first problem on the list:

Assessment ("A")	Plan ("P")
1. No records of receiving DA2PP vaccinations	1. Parvovirus ELISA snap test

The format that is selected, or any combination thereof, is largely based upon preference and will be effective as long as care is taken so that each section, the "A" and the "P," is complete.

END-OF-CHAPTER SUMMARY

The "P" in SOAP notes stands for *plan.*

The purpose of this section is to identify what measures will be taken to address, medically manage, and (ideally) resolve the patient's problem(s).

Every patient care plan has three components:

- Diagnostic recommendations
- Therapeutic recommendations
- Management recommendations or client communication notes.

These components may be listed separately under the "P" section of the SOAP note, or they may be lumped together as one. The format is less important than the contents.

Diagnostic recommendations outline patient-specific tests that the client is being advised to pursue. These may include:

- Body fluid analysis
- Imaging studies
- Exploratory surgery
- Necropsy.

Diagnostic recommendations are rarely appropriate as the sole plan for patient care. Diagnostic tests may have a turnaround time that is substantial and requires the patient to be managed while test results are pending.

Therapeutic recommendations represent a second arm of case management. These specifically address the patient's problems and target clinical signs with the intent to palliate, if not resolve, them.

Therapeutic recommendations may include:

- Prescription medications
- OTC medications, vitamins, and/or supplements
- Supportive care
- Hospitalization.

Management recommendations document what has been discussed with clients about treatment plans and patient follow-up. When will the patient return to a recheck? What steps has the client agreed to take between now and then?

References

1. Cameron S, Turtle-song I. Learning to write case notes using the SOAP format. J Couns Dev. 2002;80(3):286–292.
2. Rockett J, Lattanzio C, Christensen C. The Veterinary Technician's Guide to Writing SOAPS: A Workbook for Critical Thinking. Heyburn, Idaho: Rockett House Publishing LLC; 2013.
3. Borcherding S. Documentation Manual for Writing SOAP Notes in Occupational Therapy. 2nd ed. Thorofare, NJ: SLACK Incorporated; 2005.
4. Kettenbach G. Writing Patient/Client Notes: Ensuring Accuracy in Documentation. 4th ed. Philadelphia: F.A. Davis Company; 2004. 248 pp.
5. Kettenbach G. Writing SOAP Notes: With Patient/Client Management Formats. 3rd ed. Philadelphia: F.A. Davis Company; 2004.
6. Lorenz MD, Neer TM, Demars PL. Small Animal Medical Diagnosis. 3rd ed. Ames, Iowa: Wiley-Blackwell; 2009. xv, 502 pp.
7. IDEXX Reference Laboratories. In: IDEXX, editor. 2014. Available from: https://www.idexx.com/en/veterinary/reference-laboratories/tests-and-services/.

Chapter 8

Common Mistakes in SOAP Notes

Writing SOAP notes is a skill. Just as all other skills can be learned, so, too, can SOAP note writing. However, that does not mean that SOAP note writing always comes easily or that it can ever be perfected. Even experienced veterinarians make mistakes with record-keeping. These mistakes are more often errors of omission than true medical errors; however, either can get you into hot water if faced with a board complaint.

Because medical records, particularly SOAP notes, are one of veterinarians' best defenses against lawsuits, it is critical that we as a profession do our part to maintain their quality.(1) Some of the most frequent errors that veterinary educators and state veterinary medical boards see are outlined below in an effort to curb bad habits before they begin.

8.1 Common Errors in "S"

When a veterinarian is caring for an inpatient, a new SOAP must be created daily.(1) Depending upon how often the patient is reassessed, there may even be more than one SOAP per inpatient per day.

Despite the best of intentions to adhere to this rule and be complete, the busy and, at times, chaotic, all-hands-on-deck approach to clinical practice means that sometimes, we must play catch-up.

In the process of playing catch-up, we may sometimes choose to cut corners or take shortcuts.

Error #1: Being Vague

It is tempting, for example, to shorten the "S" of an inpatient to the following statement:

"Patient is unchanged from yesterday."

Although there may be truth to it, this statement is too vague to be helpful, particularly as time passes. You may know what this statement means relative to the patient today and maybe even tomorrow. However, 12 months from now, if you recalled this snapshot in time of this particular patient on that particular day, would you know precisely what you meant by the word *unchanged?*

Unchanged may refer to so many things, including, but not limited to:

- Activity level
- Appetite
- Attitude
- Bowel movement consistency and frequency
- Coughing
- Gait
- Mentation
- Mobility
- Pain status
- Response to medications
- Sneezing
- Tolerance towards handling
- Urine production
- Vomiting
- Diarrhea.

It may be that all of these factors are unchanged. However, truncating the patient's entire overnight experience to one word is inappropriate and undescriptive.(1, 2)

Using the word *unchanged* implies that the patient underwent a cursory examination, something we might refer to, in clinical practice, as a "drive-by" or a "once-over."

You would do better to clarify what, specifically, is *unchanged* so that it becomes clear to overseeing bodies that the patient was indeed thoroughly assessed.

Being vague also removes the opportunity for the clinician to further develop critical thinking skills.

Think of each SOAP note as an opportunity to practice problem-solving. You get out of each case as much as you invest in the SOAP note because the SOAP note is a way to process the nuances of patient health.

Error #2: Using First-Person Pronouns

A second common "S" error is to use first-person pronouns when documenting the case history. For example:

"I asked Mrs. Z____ if Fluffy could have gotten into anything, but I didn't get a resounding 'yes.' It seemed to me that she was unsure."

Using first-person pronouns in medical documentation is inappropriate because the SOAP note is intended to be written for the patient, about the patient, rather than as a monologue by the clinician.(3, 4) There is no place for "I" in a SOAP note.

Instead of inserting the first-person pronoun, "I," remove yourself from the statement altogether. A revision of the statement above is listed below:

"Owner uncertain if Fluffy got into something."

If you were using shorthand, that is, "O" for owner and "P" for patient, that same sentence might be abbreviated to:

"O uncertain if P got into something."

Error #3: Overusing Quotes

A third common error in "S" is to overuse quotes. Quotes are a way to present subjective data objectively.(4) When overused, they inefficiently capture the main points. The burden then falls upon the reader to extract key concepts, line by line, and hope not to be buried in the detail!

For instance, let us assume that the following quotes were captured during history-taking and recorded in the "S" section of the SOAP note:

- "Penny feels sick to her stomach."
- "She is smacking her lips together as if she has something sticky stuck to her mouth and can't get it off."
- "She wants to throw up – I see her belly trying to force it out of her – but she can't; nothing comes up."
- "It is not like her to turn her nose up at dinner, but she is now."

Although the reader is able to follow the comments above, they read more like a transcript. These quotes do not add anything, but bulk, to the medical record.

The essence of this clinical conversation could have been much more concisely captured by documenting the following:

"Patient is lip-smacking, with non-productive retching and inappetence."

Using shorthand, that same statement might be written as:

"P is lip-smacking, with non-productive retching and inappetence."

Quotes should be reserved for situations when legal recourse is anticipated. For example, quotes would be an appropriate means of documenting the following:

- Confessions:
  - "My boyfriend beat Fluffy until she couldn't get up."
- Defamatory statements:
  - "You are a quack."
  - "You are incompetent."
  - "You killed my dog."
- Threatening statements towards the patient:
  - "If you don't treat Fluffy for free, I will shoot her."
- Threatening statements towards you or your team:
  - "I am going to get you."
  - "You better watch your back."
  - "You will be sorry."

Error #4: Documenting Unfounded Assumptions about the Client

Veterinarians are only human.

As human beings, we may make assumptions about our clients, whether or not they are true. We may also come to inappropriate conclusions about them or judge them unfairly.

Although best kept to ourselves, these statements may erroneously trickle into the medical record.

There is no room in the medical record for statements such as:

- "The client is a lush."
- "The client is cheap."
- "The client is incompetent."
- "The client is mentally unstable."

Unfortunately, the author has read these statements and many more in colleagues' medical records.

These statements are inappropriate.

It may be true that the client is cheap, incompetent, or mentally unstable.

However, the first two descriptions are judgmental and therefore unnecessary.

The third description is beyond our area of expertise. Veterinarians are not mental health experts. It is not within our purview to diagnose patients with mental instability or to suggest that they may be mentally unsound.

It would be best to avoid making judgments altogether and instead focus on actions rather than personal habits or behaviors.

If a client appears to be drunk and this impacts the outcome of the case, then it is appropriate to document actions that prompted this conclusion. For example, you might write that:

- "The client was inarticulate."
- "The client was slurring her words."
- "The client was ataxic."
- "The client appeared to be confused and asked, 'Where am I?' multiple times."

8.2 Common Errors in "O"

Although Chapter 1 emphasized brevity in medical documentation, there are times during veterinary consultations when details are essential.

To be comprehensive, the "O" section of the SOAP note must be detailed. It must describe the patient's physical examination findings in sufficient detail so that if the reader were to close his eyes and imagine the patient, he would be able to accurately recreate the lesions in his mind.

Unfortunately, the "O" section of the SOAP note rarely provides the level of detail that is required.

Consider the following phrases that are commonly listed as physical examination abnormalities:

- Aural discharge
- Ocular discharge
- Nasal discharge.

When there are paired structures, the veterinarian may fail to document which structure is affected.

- Are both ears, eyes, and nasal passageways involved?

Furthermore, what specifically is abnormal about these structures?
Discharge is not a very specific term.

- Is there *serous* discharge?
- Is there mucus?
- Is the discharge wet or dry?
- Is the discharge transparent or opaque?
- Is the discharge colored?

All of these adjectives paint a picture. Without these adjectives, it is very difficult to envision what the record-keeper saw on physical examination.

Vagueness with regards to discharge quality and consistency is common. In addition, vagueness is also often associated with the following paired structures:

- Forelimbs
  - "The patient has forelimb lameness."
    - fatal flaw: *which* forelimb?
- Hind limbs
  - "The patient has hind limb lameness."
    - fatal flaw: *which* hind limb?
- Lymph nodes
  - "All lymph nodes were normal."
    - fatal flaw: *which* ones?
      - *which* ones were felt?
      - *which* should be felt?
      - what does *normal* mean?
      - does *normal* refer to size, shape, texture, or symmetry?

- Paws

  - "The patient is non-weight bearing on his paw."

    - fatal flaw: *which* paw?

Clinicians are also sometimes vague about body parts or regions of the body. For instance, they may document within the "O" section of the SOAP note that the patient had "papulopustular lesions."

This is a great description of what the lesions look like in this specific patient.

However, the same description fails to establish where the rash is on the body.

To the writer, the description makes sense in the moment. S/he can picture the patient and the lesions. S/he knows what s/he means when writing that statement.

Unfortunately, his/her memory will fade. When it does, who will remember the location of the lesions?

It is better to include geographical location in the description now so that there is no room for uncertainty later.

When describing skin lesions, it is particularly important to be detailed. Consider the following descriptors that should be included in the medical record:

- Number of lesions
- Size of lesions
- Shapes of lesions
- Color(s) of lesions
- Surface of lesions:

  - rounded or domed
  - flat or plaque-like

- Distribution of lesions:

  - isolated
  - clustered.

Photographs can help enormously, particularly when skin lesions are involved.

Photographs can also play an important role in facilitating comparisons of patient progress, between the initial visit and today's recheck.

Not every veterinarian has access to electronic medical record (EMR) software that supports image uploads.

That being said, even if uploads are possible, what if those images were inadvertently deleted?

Would you remember how to describe the lesions that you witnessed in the examination room?

Would you be able to conjure up an image from what is inside of your head?

If the answer is no, then you really need to provide a thorough account in writing of what you saw and how it changed over time.

8.3 Common Errors in "A"

Recall that Chapter 6 reviewed the problem list and emphasized the importance of being complete. All problems are listed, even those that do not appear to be related to the primary problem, in order of their severity and/or urgency, from most to least.

A common mistake in the "A" section of the SOAP note is failure to prioritize the problem list so that minor problems precede major problems.

If the "A" section becomes a "blenderized" version of all problems, great and small, then it becomes that much more challenging to streamline the "P" section. The result is a jumbled plan that skips around in an illogical manner.

Recall, for example, the case of the 2-year-old, male intact (MI) Rottweiler dog. Under the dog's "A" section, 17 problems were listed. These problems were prioritized.

What if that had not been the case? What if priorities had not been outlined and the very first problem listed was the behavioral issue of cat chasing?

A cursory glance at an improperly prioritized record may lead to the erroneous assumption that the patient is stable. In fact, this patient required immediate medical intervention.

8.4 Common Errors in "P"

Chapter 7 addressed the importance of being detail-oriented when discussing the administration of medications as part of the therapeutic plan. That attention to detail is equally important when it comes to planning next steps, including the next visit.

The number of patients who are lost to follow-up every year is astronomical. We would like to think that this is because the patient's health significantly improved in the client's estimation and the client felt that a recheck examination was unnecessary.

However, how many times does a patient *not* return according to our time schedule, only to present for a recheck examination at a later point in time, frustrated because the clinical signs have recurred?

How many times does a puppy or kitten have to restart their vaccination series because they missed a booster?

How many times must we re-prescribe antibiotics because they were discontinued prematurely or they were not given at all?

It is easy for the clinician to cast blame on the client. How many times have you heard the phrase, *if they had just listened . . .!*

The reality is that clients only hear a fraction of what is said. Studies in human medicine demonstrate that patients frequently do not recall what they are told at time of discharge and/or do not always fully understand what is shared with them.(5–8)

The tendency to incompletely hear or understand medical recommendations adversely impacts client compliance and satisfaction with healthcare.(9–11)

Because clients hear only a fraction of what is said, it is critical that we make clear recommendations that are emphasized verbally and in writing.

Discharge statements must include follow-up instructions that are specific. Concerning follow-up, discharge statements should answer the following questions:

- When should follow-up occur?

  - tonight
  - tomorrow
  - 72 hours
  - next week
  - next month
  - before the antibiotics run out
  - after the antibiotics run out
  - in six months
  - next year

- How should follow-up occur?

  - by email
  - by telephone
  - by text
  - in person

- Who is going to initiate follow-up?

  - the client
  - the receptionist
  - the veterinary technician
  - the veterinarian

- Which events require follow-up to take place sooner than anticipated?

  - if the patient is not keeping medication down
  - if the patient is not eating 24–48 hours from now
  - if the patient has two or more seizures within the next 24 hours
  - if the patient's resting respiratory rate exceeds 30 breaths per minute
  - if the patient vomits more than three times overnight.

If we do not specify what we want for our patients, then how can we expect our clients to follow through?

Clients may be perceptive when it comes to their pets' health and well-being, but they are not mind readers. Nor should we expect them to be.

Be specific when verbalizing recommendations and explain *why* those recommendations need to be followed. It is even more important to put those recommendations in writing. That way, if questions arise between now and the next visit, you or any other member of the veterinary team that reviews the record can reiterate what the next steps are, and when, where, how, and why they are needed.

END-OF-CHAPTER SUMMARY

Writing SOAP notes can be challenging, even for seasoned veterinarians.

SOAP note errors are common.

If a case is brought before a state board of veterinary medical examiners or another supervising body, SOAP note errors can result in violations.

SOAP note errors can be the reason for a veterinarian losing a lawsuit.

Remember the adage: it didn't happen if it isn't written.

In other words, documentation is key, and proper documentation begins with SOAP notes.

It behooves veterinarians to work towards improving the quality of their SOAP notes because SOAP notes constitute a significant part of the medical record, and the medical record is a legal document.

Common SOAP note errors are broken down by section (S, O, A, and P) and include:

- Vagueness or lack of details
    - "patient is unchanged from yesterday"
        - what does *unchanged* mean?
    - "all lymph nodes were normal"
        - which lymph nodes does *all* refer to? Truly, which were palpable?
    - "nasal discharge"
        - what is the consistency and color of the discharge?
        - from one or both nares?
    - "papulopustular lesions"
        - where? Diffusely or regionally distributed?
    - "swollen paw"
        - *which* paw?
    - unfounded assumptions about the client
        - "the client doesn't care"
        - "the client is unstable."

To reduce common SOAP note errors:

- Be specific
    - when and how should follow-up occur? Who will initiate it?

- Document threatening statements or client confessions
- Document actions rather than behaviors
- Identify

  - number, size, shape, color, and distribution of lesions.

References

1. Wilson JF. Law and Ethics of the Veterinary Profession. Yardley, PA: Priority Press, Ltd.; 2000.
2. Fleenor J. SOAP Notes: The Down and Dirty on Squeaky Clean Documentation. Denver, CO: shift 4 publishing, LLC; 2007.
3. Kettenbach G. Writing SOAP Notes: With Patient/Client Management Formats. 3rd ed. Philadelphia: F.A. Davis Company; 2004.
4. Borcherding S. Documentation Manual for Writing SOAP Notes in Occupational Therapy. 2nd ed. Thorofare, NJ: SLACK Incorporated; 2005.
5. Zeng-Treitler Q, Kim H, Hunter M. Improving patient comprehension and recall of discharge instructions by supplementing free texts with pictographs. AMIA Annu Symp Proc. 2008:849–853.
6. Heng KW, Tham KY, How KY, Foo JS, Lau YH, Li AY. Recall of discharge advice given to patients with minor head injury presenting to a Singapore emergency department. Singapore Med J. 2007;48(12):1107–1110.
7. Hwang SW, Tram CQ, Knarr N. The effect of illustrations on patient comprehension of medication instruction labels. BMC Fam Pract. 2005;6(1):26.
8. Spandorfer JM, Karras DJ, Hughes LA, Caputo C. Comprehension of discharge instructions by patients in an urban emergency department. Ann Emerg Med. 1995;25(1):71–74.
9. Clark PA, Drain M, Gesell SB, Mylod DM, Kaldenberg DO, Hamilton J. Patient perceptions of quality in discharge instruction. Patient Educ Couns. 2005;59(1):56–68.
10. Clarke C, Friedman SM, Shi K, Arenovich T, Monzon J, Culligan C. Emergency department discharge instructions comprehension and compliance study. CJEM. 2005;7(1):5–11.
11. Watt D, Wertzler W, Brannan G. Patient expectations of emergency department care: phase I–a focus group study. CJEM. 2005;7(1):12–16.

Chapter 9

Academic SOAP Notes

Chapters 4–8 reviewed the *clinical* SOAP note. The *clinical* SOAP note is intended for use in everyday practice and by veterinary students as they advance to the clinical years of their curriculum.

The *clinical* SOAP note assumes a basic understanding of the pathophysiology of disease.

Let us remind ourselves of the differential diagnoses for vomiting that were outlined in Chapter 6 concerning the case of the 2-year-old, male intact (MI) Rottweiler dog:

- Neoplasia
    - gastrointestinal lymphoma
- Infectious
    - parvovirus
    - bacterial gastroenteritis
    - leptospirosis
- Toxicities
    - ethylene glycol ingestion
- Structural
    - intussusception
    - pyloric stenosis
- Congenital
    - hiatal hernia
- Other
    - foreign body
    - dysautonomia

- Metabolic
    - hypoadrenocorticism
    - pancreatitis
    - hepatitis
    - gastritis
    - gastroenteritis
- Parasitic
    - roundworms
    - whipworms
    - hookworms
    - tapeworms
    - *Giardia*
- Diet
    - dietary indiscretion
    - food sensitivity
    - food allergy
- Husbandry
    - see diet.

Note how the differential diagnoses have been listed without establishing the link to the primary problem, vomiting.

The *clinical* SOAP assumes that these links are understood. That is, for the writer of the SOAP note to compile the list of differential diagnoses, s/he presumably had to review the pathophysiology of each relative to the primary problem.

For a seasoned clinician, this process comes second nature. It is as automatic as tying a surgeon's knot.

However, for the novice, it presents a challenge.

Every day on the clinic floor, the novice is presented with "firsts" – first case of hemorrhagic gastroenteritis, first case of splenic torsion, first case of pancreatitis, first case of hepatic adenocarcinoma, and so on.

Unless the novice has firsthand experience of these conditions, s/he lacks the clinical acumen to include them as differential diagnoses.

Differential diagnoses are, in a sense, too specific to come up with on one's own, without prior knowledge or training in the diagnosis of each particular disease state.

So, unless the novice memorizes clinical algorithms for particular disease presentations or plays the game of "Dr. Google," searching online for causes of clinical signs in the patient, it is too great a leap for the novice to jump from problem to differential.

A bridge must be connected from A to B. The *academic* SOAP bridges the gap.(1, 2)

Think of the *academic* SOAP as an exercise to train the novice how to think like a seasoned veterinarian. The exercise requires the novice to consider the underlying mechanism(s) by which each problem on the problem list came about.

This allows the novice to refresh his/her memory of anatomy, physiology, pathology, and pathophysiology in order to come up with big picture concepts of what may have led to the disease state.

Initially, these concepts are quite broad. However, as the student matures, s/he funnels down to the details that lead to a set of appropriate, narrowed differential diagnoses. (1, 2)

Consider a partially written SOAP note for a case example involving a MI, domestic shorthaired (DSH) kitten:

"S"

Found along street corner in Good Samaritan's neighborhood. Good Samaritan thought patient (P) was deceased until he approached and heard a mew. P covered in fleas. Did not resist being placed in the car and brought to the clinic. Unknown past medical history.

"O"

T: 103.6°F	BCS: 2/9
P: 186 beats per minute (bpm)	MCS: 1/3: moderate muscle loss
R: 68 breaths per minute	PCV: 8% (25–41%)
Weight: 0.9 kg/2.0 lb	

General appearance (GA): quiet, alert, sluggish to respond to touch.

Integument (INTEG): moderate skin tenting; entire coat crawling with fleas; marked amount of flea dirt diffusely peppering coat, but concentrated at tail base; P is intermittently pruritic when combed. Removed five attached ticks between bridge of nose and ears; removed two more from the nape of the neck.

Eyes/ears/nose/throat (EENT): "cauliflower" scarring of external pinna AS with narrowed external ear canal AS; negative for gross aural debris; non-erythematous; unable to visualize either tympanic membrane.

Cardiovascular/respiratory (CV/RESP): Grade 2/6 parasternal, systolic murmur; pale pink, tacky mucous membranes; tachycardic; tachypneic.

Gastrointestinal (GI): diffusely doughy abdomen on palpation – unable to palpate feces in descending colon; small bowel palpates as being empty but of apparently normal thickness.

Urogenital (URO): small, supple urinary bladder; both kidneys palpate as smooth-surfaced and symmetrical; non-reactive on palpation of either.

Lymphatic (LN): bilaterally symmetrical, palpable submandibular, prescapular, and popliteal lymph nodes; unable to appreciate axillary or inguinal lymph nodes.

Musculoskeletal (MS): moderate muscle loss – bilaterally symmetrical; whole body weak.

Nervous (NEURO): subdued/delayed mentation.

"A"

1. Severe anemia
2. Flea infestation
3. Tick infestation
4. Grade 2/6 parasternal, systolic murmur
5. Tachycardic
6. Tachypneic
7. Moderate muscle loss
8. Doughy feel to abdomen
9. Unknown vaccination history
10. Unknown serological status
11. Scarring of external pinna AS with narrowing of associated external ear canal.

In a *clinical* SOAP, the next step would be to pair the aforementioned problems with differential diagnoses as outlined in Chapter 6.

The seasoned veterinarian should easily be able to connect the dots between ectoparasite infestation and anemia. Flea bite anemia and/or cytauxzoonosis must be top considerations.

The kitten's unknown serological status makes feline leukemia virus (FeLV) and/or feline immunodeficiency virus (FIV) possible.

The kitten's unthrifty, underweight state and presumptive poor diet are likely contributing factors.

Due to experience, the case is easily solved.

However, the case may not be as clear-cut and dry to a novice, who is just beginning to make use of critical thinking skills to navigate veterinary medicine on a case-by-case basis.

The novice may consider fleas as a probable cause of anemia, but may be significantly less familiar with the other differential diagnoses.

Rather than expect the novice to make that leap overnight, the *academic* SOAP provides the novice with the opportunity to take baby steps, to explore the problem of anemia one step at a time until the mystery is progressively unraveled.(2)

The *academic* SOAP has the novice begin by asking the following question:

"What are the major causes of anemia?"

The answer to this question is not a differential diagnosis. The answer is a process – more than one, actually.

The broad causes of anemia are: (3, 4)

- Blood loss
- Decreased production of erythrocytes (red blood cells or RBCs)
- Increased destruction of erythrocytes.

This is the first layer of the *academic* SOAP under the problem of anemia in the "A" section. It may be the furthest that a first-year veterinary student is expected to reach, depending upon the curriculum to which s/he is exposed.

As the student advances through the curriculum and the gaps in knowledge are filled in, more layers of information emerge.

For example, the second layer of the *academic* SOAP under the problem of anemia in the "A" section will expand upon each process that leads to anemia: (3, 4)

- Blood loss:

  - external blood loss

    - blood-sucking ectoparasites
    - epistaxis
    - hematochezia
    - hematuria
    - hemoptysis
    - melena

- internal blood loss

  - blood-sucking endoparasites
  - internal organ injury due to

    - being hit by a car
    - spontaneous rupture, as from splenic hemangiosarcoma

- Decreased production of red blood cells can stem from:

  - primary bone marrow disease:

    - the progenitor cells for red blood cells reside in the bone marrow
    - if these cells become dysfunctional, as in the case of aplastic anemia, new red blood cells are not produced to replace those that have completed their lifespan
    - over time, the population of mature red blood cells in the bloodstream declines, causing anemia

  - renal disease:

    - the kidney is responsible for producing erythropoietin, which is responsible for stimulating the bone marrow to produce new red blood cells
    - if the kidney is failing, as in chronic renal disease, less erythropoietin is produced
    - less produced erythropoietin means less stimulation of the bone marrow
    - over time, the population of mature red blood cells in the bloodstream declines, causing anemia

  - poor diet:

    - in order to produce new red blood cells, the body needs sufficient levels of iron, folate, and vitamin B12
    - without adequate nutrition, levels of these necessary ingredients may remain too low to adequately produce new red blood cells
    - over time, the population of mature red blood cells in the bloodstream declines, causing anemia

- Increased destruction of red blood cells can stem from:

  - autoimmune disease, such as hemolytic anemia

    - in hemolytic anemia, the body loses recognition of self versus non-self
    - the result is that the body attacks its own red blood cells
    - over time, the population of mature red blood cells in the bloodstream declines, causing anemia

  - diseases of the spleen

    - one of the spleen's everyday functions is to filter worn-out blood cells from the circulation

- if the spleen becomes enlarged or diseased, it may filter too many red blood cells, causing a decline in the number of circulating erythrocytes
- over time, the population of mature red blood cells in the bloodstream declines, causing anemia.

The final layer of the *academic* SOAP under the problem of anemia in the "A" section arises from those critical thinking skills that allow us to prioritize which conceptual ideas are most likely to be valid differential diagnoses.

Another way to think about this layer is to weigh the options and decide which avenue is most likely for that particular patient. For example: (3, 4)

- Decreased production of red blood cells can stem from:
  - primary bone marrow disease:

    Bone marrow disease in a kitten is highly unlikely.

  - renal disease:

    Although renal disease cannot be ruled out without performing a serum bio-chemistry panel and urinalysis, it would be expected to produce additional clinical signs that were not noted here.

    It is true that the kitten is not owned, and therefore the Good Samaritan may not have witnessed these clinical signs.

    However, I would have expected to see the following physical examination findings if the kitten did in fact have renal disease of this severity: uremic breath, bilaterally small kidneys (if chronic renal disease) versus bilaterally enlarged kidneys (if acute renal failure as from a toxin). That being said, acute renal failure does not typically result in peracute anemia.

  - poor diet:

    Cannot be ruled out as a contributing factor, given the patient's unknown health history, current status as a stray, poor body condition score, and poor muscle condition score.

    The patient's unthrifty state suggests that he is malnourished.

- Increased destruction of red blood cells can stem from:
  - autoimmune disease, which is highly unlikely in a kitten
  - diseases of the spleen, which are highly unlikely in a kitten

- Blood loss
  - external blood loss

    There is significant evidence that the patient is infested with blood-sucking ectoparasites.

Flea infestation can cause appreciable anemia, particularly in kittens, and ticks can also result in cytauxzoonosis.

This cause of anemia is strongly supported by physical examination findings.

- internal blood loss

  Infection with blood-sucking endoparasites cannot be ruled out as an additional cause of blood loss.

Appreciate that this unfolding of the *academic* SOAP in bite-sized pieces allows students to build onto their foundation of knowledge as it grows substantially during their preclinical years.

The structure of the *academic* SOAP also allows students to identify so-called learning issues: gaps in their knowledge base that could benefit from additional study.

Students can be encouraged to take an active role in the learning process by researching these areas and reporting back to the veterinary team and/or the attending clinician at rounds the following day.

The following are examples of learning issues that may have arisen from the exercise above, involving the anemic kitten:

- What is the average life span of an erythrocyte?
- What is the process by which erythrocytes mature in the bone marrow?
- How precisely are damaged erythrocytes removed from circulation by the spleen?
- How exactly does erythropoietin trigger the bone marrow to produce new erythrocytes?
- Other than a decreased packed cell volume (PCV), how else is anemia reflected in the complete blood count (CBC)?
- What is the role of iron in erythrocyte formation?
- How does a deficiency in vitamin B12 lead to anemia?
- What is the most appropriate medical management for this patient?
- When is it appropriate to consider a blood transfusion?
- What are the risks associated with transfusing blood from one cat to another?
- What are feline blood types?
- Are major and minor cross matches necessary prior to transfusing a feline patient?
- What avenues are available to treat the ectoparasite infestations?
- What is the mechanism of action for each flea and tick preventative?
- In addition to flea bite anemia, which infectious diseases could the patient contract from the fleas and/or ticks?
- What is the resting energy requirement (RER) for this patient?
- How many calories are required for this patient to maintain weight?
- How many calories are required for this patient to gain weight?
- What is refeeding syndrome and do you need to consider this syndrome for this patient?

By actively engaging in the acquisition of new knowledge, students are more likely to retain practical information that they will need to recall in clinical rotations and beyond.

Creating links between coursework and seeing how one classroom topic is interwoven with another sets the stage for higher levels of learning, which will bolster critical thinking and problem-solving.

Veterinary students should be encouraged to go through the process of creating *academic* SOAPs for every case that they see. Case-based classroom exercises are an ideal way for students to get involved with SOAP writing early in the curriculum.

One additional, minor difference between the *clinical* and *academic* SOAP is that the latter often begins with a summary statement.(2)

This case summary precedes the "S" and typically includes the signalment and presenting complaint as demonstrated by the following examples:

- "Darcy is a 6-year-old female spayed (FS) Golden Retriever dog that presents for a three-day history of anorexia."
- "Otis is an 8-year-old male castrated (MC) Pug dog that presents for a two-day history of scooting and excessive perineal grooming."
- "Juniper is a 16-year-old mare Quarter Horse that presents for a Coggins test prior to interstate travel."
- "Bella is a 7-year-old FS Himalayan cat that presents for a five-day recheck of a superficial corneal ulcer OD."

The case summary statement provides context and a framework for building the rest of the SOAP note.

The case summary also teaches students how to introduce a case to the veterinary team and provides a starting point for students to invite case discussions at rounds.

END-OF-CHAPTER SUMMARY

Chapters 4–8 reviewed the process of writing the *clinical* SOAP note. The *clinical* SOAP note is an important part of the medical record in clinical practice.

Clinical SOAP notes are abbreviated in that they assume a basic level of understanding concerning the pathophysiology of disease. For example, if gastrointestinal lymphoma is listed as a differential diagnosis for vomiting in a canine patient in the "A" section, the *clinical* SOAP note assumes that the clinician understands the link between lymphoma and the clinical sign.

The *academic* SOAP note is a training exercise that veterinary students can use to clarify the link between clinical signs and active disease processes. In a sense, the *academic* SOAP can be thought of as a bridge between didactic classroom learning and the experiential learning that takes place on the clinic floor. When students write *academic* SOAP notes, they have to consider the mechanisms that underlie clinical signs. This involves integration between veterinary disciplines, particularly anatomy, physiology, pathology, and pathophysiology.

First-year students tend to think in terms of broad concepts. For instance, the clinical sign of pallor may trigger a differential diagnosis list that includes anemia. Because students at this level of the curriculum have not typically been taught internal medicine and pathology, their understanding of anemia is quite elementary. When asked to consider what causes anemia in veterinary patients, three broad possibilities may come to mind:

- Blood loss, as in hemorrhage
- Decreased erythrocyte (RBC) production
- Increased erythrocyte destruction.

These broad categories represent the first layer of understanding concerning the differential diagnosis of anemia.

As students expand their knowledge, they are able to create the second layer. For example, they may learn that decreased erythrocyte production may stem from:

- Dietary deficiency
- Primary bone marrow disease
- Renal disease.

Step by step, layer by layer, students' understanding of anemia creates a comprehensive list of rule-outs. This list thoroughly describes each process, how it relates to the clinical sign of interest, and how likely it is to be a causative agent.

In this way, the academic SOAP note nourishes the skill of critical thinking to optimize case management.

References

1. Lane I. The Problem Oriented Medical Approach. Available from: http://libguides.utk.edu/ld.php?content_id=7167021
2. Gardner H, Hines S. The Academic SOAP: A Beginner's Guide to Help You Get Started. Washington: Washington State University. Available from: https://www.vetmed.wsu.edu/docs/librariesprovider16/docs---diagnostic-challenge/soap_beginnners-guide.pdf?sfvrsn=0
3. Côté E. Clinical Veterinary Advisor. Dogs and Cats. 3rd ed. St. Louis, MO: Elsevier Mosby; 2015. xxxvii, 1642 pp.
4. Ettinger SJ, Feldman EC, Côté E. Textbook of Veterinary Internal Medicine: Diseases of the Dog and the Cat. 8th ed. St. Louis, MO: Elsevier; 2017.

Chapter 10

Variations of SOAP Notes

10.1 "Herd Health" SOAP Notes

Up to this point in the text, SOAP notes have been described as a way to document healthcare for a single patient.

However, veterinary medicine is unique as a profession because it often requires clinicians to deal with more than one patient at a time, particularly in situations involving "herd health."

We often consider herd health in the context of cattle. However, herd health is a much broader term that could include:

- Bands of wild horses
- Litters of puppies or kittens
- Collections of zoo animals, such as a colony of prairie dogs.

Cases involving "herd health" still require SOAP notes.

So how then do we go about writing a SOAP note for more than one patient?

The framework of the "herd health" SOAP note remains the same: there is still an "S," an "O," an "A," and a "P."

Each section includes the same content that was described in Chapters 4–7.

The key difference is that rather than SOAPing the problems of one individual, problems are SOAPed with regards to the herd.(1)

For example, the "S" section of the SOAP note for a herd of dairy cattle will typically emphasize the environment in which the herd is maintained, as well as key management and facilities operations that might be relevant to the primary problem.

In a situation involving calf diarrhea, so-called scours, the "S" section of the SOAP note will likely emphasize:

- How the calves are housed

  - group housing
  - individual calf hutches
  - isolation wards

- How many calves appear to be affected out of the total number of calves at that facility
- When the clinical signs began
- How the clinical signs have progressed.

In a situation involving potential abortion storms in a dairy herd, the "S" section of the SOAP note will likely emphasize:

- How many cows have aborted
- At what stage(s) of pregnancy have they aborted
- When specifically the cows aborted in terms of dates and in relation to one another
- How many cows have since returned to estrus
- How the cows were bred

  - natural cover
  - artificial insemination

- Vaccination history

  - before breeding
  - during pregnancy

- On-site biosecurity

  - which people (if any) are allowed to visit the farm and, if so, when?
  - is there a protocol for visitors to interact with cattle?
  - what is the protocol for visitors to interact with cattle?
  - which people (if any) have left the farm to visit other farms, and when, relative to the abortions?
  - have any cattle from the farm left the premises and returned?
  - is there a protocol for dealing with cattle that return to the farm?
  - what is the protocol for cattle that return to the farm?
  - have any new cows been introduced to the herd and, if so, when?

The "O" section of the SOAP note for a herd typically describes the physical examination findings of the affected patients only – specifically, those that were examined by the veterinarian when s/he visited the ranch.(1)

The veterinarian may conclude in the "O," for example, that 3 of 31 cows have mastitis or that 24 out of 62 cows are open.

The "A" section of the SOAP note for "herd health" cases is similar to the "A" section of the SOAP note for individual patients. However, in addition to listing problems that individual animals have within the herd, the "A" section of the SOAP note may also include herd-level problems, such as:

- Inappropriate vaccination strategies
- Poor biosecurity.

Likewise, the "P" section of the SOAP note for "herd health" cases is likely to include strategies for resolving clinical signs within the herd or risk management decisions for the entire operation.

Examples of statements that might appear in the "P" section of the SOAP note for "herd health" cases include:

- Improve biosecurity by discontinuing tours of the farm by the local school district
- Change the teat dipping protocols for the dairy to reduce the risk of mastitis
- Increase the protein content of the formula that is fed to the calves
- Reduce the ambient temperature in the barn by installing floor and ceiling fans.

10.2 Other Versions of SOAP Notes

SOAP notes are considered the standard by which record-keeping is maintained at most private practices and teaching hospitals.

What has been presented here, for both individual patients and "herd health" consultations, are two formats that you are most likely to see as veterinary students and as practicing clinicians.

Understand that these formats vary somewhat depending upon the setting (companion animal vs. ambulatory) and the practice's preferences.

That being said, you will find that there is very little difference in content between the SOAP note at Practice A and the SOAP note at Practice B, or between the SOAP note at Specialty Service A and the SOAP note at Specialty Service B.

The primary differences, by and large, boil down to the style.

As a veterinary student, do not get caught up in these differences. Take note of what each service, specialty service, clinical rotation, and practice prefers and adapt to their approach.

Learn the strengths and styles of each clinician you work with until you graduate and develop the confidence to construct your own system.

Over time, SOAP notes will continue to evolve. Whether their structure will continue to borrow from human healthcare remains to be seen. However, as physicians develop new approaches to case management, veterinarians may follow suit.

For instance, there has been a relatively recent trend in human medicine to convert the once standard SOAP notes into SOAPS notes. SOAPS notes have an additional "S" that stands for *safety*.

This second "S" arose from the mandate from accrediting bodies in human healthcare that medical residencies incorporate patient safety into the curriculum.(2)

SOAPS was one proposed solution.

By integrating the second "S" into medical documentation, physicians are required to consider safety as part of every patient's case management. The hope is that doing so will prevent safety from being overlooked, which may translate into fewer preventable deaths per year.(2)

Items that could be included in this second "S" are:

- Action plans for use in the veterinary teaching hospital
  - examples:
    - "Pad the patient's kennel as a precaution in the event of a seizure."
    - "Calculate an emergency dose of epinephrine in the event that the patient codes."
    - "Remove IV catheter prior to discharging patient from the hospital."
- Action plans for at-home use by the veterinary client
  - examples:
    - "Alert owner that a baby gate must be placed to block off the stairs because the patient is at risk of falling down them due to its current state of unsteadiness."
    - "Tell owner to remove the patient's bandage on the right forelimb as soon as she arrives home."

To the author's knowledge, SOAPS has not yet been adapted for use in veterinary medicine, nor has it become standard practice in human healthcare.

However, it is an approach that is worth considering given that veterinary practices are not immune to medical error.

END-OF-CHAPTER SUMMARY

Through Chapter 9 of this text, SOAP notes have been discussed as they pertain to the management of a single patient.

However, many facets of veterinary medicine are unique in that they require the documentation of care for multiples of animals.

Historically, this aspect of veterinary medicine has been referred to as "herd health."

When we hear the term "herd health," situations involving production animal medicine tend to come to mind. For example, management of:

- Dairy and beef herds
- Swine
- Flocks of sheep and goats
- Flocks of fowl.

"Herd health" may also be used to describe bands of wild horses, such as Mustangs in the grassland regions of the western United States.

"Herd health" is equally appropriate for discussions on collections of wildlife at zoos and aquariums.

"Herd health" may even be used to consider groups of companion animal patients, although we often do not think of them as such:

- Temporary residents of animal shelters
- Litters of puppies and kittens.

When we write SOAP notes for these collections of animals, we use the same structure: S, O, A, and P.

What differs is that rather than SOAPing the problems of one individual, problems are SOAPed with regards to the herd. For example, the history portion of the SOAP note, the "S," will likely include numbers of animals affected: 3/31 cows have mastitis and 14 are off feed.

The "P" portion of the SOAP note will also emphasize strategies for resolving clinical signs within the herd or risk management decisions for the entire operation.

SOAP notes are likely to continue to evolve. For example, to encourage healthcare providers to consider patient safety, some medical schools have advocated changing SOAP notes into SOAPS. The second "S" stands for *safety*. It is hoped that SOAPS will reduce medical errors and improve patient outcomes.

References

1. Gardner H, Hines S. The Academic SOAP: A Beginner's Guide to Help You Get Started. Washington: Washington State University. Available from: https://www.vetmed.wsu.edu/docs/librariesprovider16/docs---diagnostic-challenge/soap_beginnners-guide.pdf?sfvrsn=0
2. Weiss PM, Lara-Torre E, Murchison AB, Spotswood L. Expanding the SOAP note to SOAPS (with S for safety): a new era in real-time safety education. J Grad Med Educ. 2009;1(2):316–318.

Chapter 11

Other Medical Documents

Chapters 4–10 introduced you to the SOAP note. SOAP notes contribute a substantial amount of documentation to every patient file.

For example, a 16-year-old Himalayan cat that presents to one clinic, once per year, for every year of its life, will have a 16-entry medical record, with 16 comprehensive SOAP notes, one per visit.

By comparison, a patient that presents for acute illness as well as wellness visits will have a lot more entries!

It is easy to appreciate how rapidly the medical record expands.

However, it is important to understand that record-keeping in veterinary medicine is not just about documenting office visits, in sickness and in health. Although these consultations set the stage for case management, veterinarians engage in additional professional activities that require written documentation. These documents supplement the patient's medical record and include:

- Operative reports
- Discharge statements
- Referral letters
- Email correspondence.

There are no universal guidelines for medical record add-ons.(1) Their structure and format varies widely between veterinarians and among practices. What one veterinarian may choose to do in a primary care setting may differ from a colleague. What is standard at one university may not be standard elsewhere.

Veterinary educators look to accrediting bodies for guidance in terms of *what* to teach. However, ultimately the institution decides *how* to instruct. Students are therefore exposed to an assortment of styles and approaches that they must learn how to make sense of over time.

What is presented here may vary from what you have seen in class or what you may have experienced on the clinic floor. Recall from past sections of this text that there is no one right approach. Medical documentation is about learning what to include and why, in a way that makes the most sense to you.

This chapter presents one approach that you may find helpful when trying to complete these medical record "extras."

11.1 Operative Reports

Just as medical case management is recorded in SOAP notes, operative reports are the means by which surgeons document surgical events.(2–4)

Operative reports in human healthcare date back to the late 1800s.(5) These early reports detailed the procedure and the anesthetic agent, but were disassociated from the patient by omitting his/her name.(3, 5)

As healthcare became organized in the 20th century, the content of these notes evolved.(3) Patients were eventually linked to procedures in order to maintain a record of what was done, to whom, in what way, and with which anticipated consequences. This allowed doctors to follow up on adverse events.(3)

Today, there are guidelines for operative reports in human healthcare at both the institutional and national level.(2, 6, 7)

In the United States (U.S.), the Joint Commission on Accreditation of Healthcare Organizations provides standards that must be upheld at all accredited institutions.(6)

In the United Kingdom (U.K.), surgical standards are under the purview of statutory bodies such as the Royal College of Surgeons (RCS). In 2008, the RCS compiled these standards into one comprehensive manual.(7) This collection outlines how to be consistent in surgical reporting to ensure patient safety and defend against litigation.(3, 8, 9)

Compliance with guidelines is also essential for correct coding of data, which is the primary way that the human healthcare industry is paid. Insurance companies rely upon codes to calculate reimbursement and to protect against fraudulent charges.(9, 10)

Incomplete operative notes result in coding errors that delay or reduce reimbursement.(9, 10) In worst case scenarios, reimbursement for surgical procedures can be denied.(9)

The human healthcare industry is under immense pressure to conform to standards so that reimbursement is expedient and meets expectations for what any given procedure is worth.

Veterinary insurance has existed worldwide since the early 1900s, and in the U.S. since 1982.(11)

Today, the North American Pet Health Insurance Association (NAPHIA) represents greater than 20 brands of insurance that are marketed throughout the U.S. and Canada. (11) As of 2015, over 1.4 million pets were insured in the U.S. alone.(12) Yet, that represents just 1% of owned pets in the United States.(13) Despite the fact that the care of companion animals alone is a billion dollar industry(14), pet insurance has been slow to take off.

Europe has taken to pet health insurance more so than in the U.S. Estimates suggest that 40% of pets are insured in England and 60% in Sweden.(15) Still, the public's perception and acceptance of veterinary insurance varies widely. A major barrier to its adoption is lack of information or misinformation.(15) Clients (and veterinarians!) do not always understand what is covered and whether the benefit of insurance exceeds the expense.(15)

Because most veterinary patients are not insured, veterinarians do not need to rely upon operative reports to justify charges on billable accounts. As a result, the veterinary industry is under less pressure than human healthcare to adopt standards for operative reports.

There is a paucity of information in the veterinary medical literature on how to create operative reports, let alone standardize them.

The American Animal Hospital Association (AAHA) comes the closest by providing surgical standards for accredited U.S. practices.(16) However, these pertain more to the maintenance of the surgical suite and surgical attire than to postoperative written documentation.(16)

To learn how to construct operative reports, the veterinary medical profession must largely rely upon human healthcare guides.

In accordance with the most current manual by the RCS, *Good Surgical Practice*, surgeons in the human medical field are required to include the following in their operative reports:(7)

- Date/time/name of procedure
- Surgeon's name/assistant's name/anesthesiologist's name
- Description of incision: i.e. size, location
- Operative findings and diagnosis
- Description of procedure
- Additional procedures performed
- Complications during procedure(s)
- Description of closure: i.e. suture material, suture size
- Estimate of blood loss
- Antibiotic prophylaxis (where applicable)
- Deep vein thrombosis (DVT) prophylaxis, where applicable
- Postoperative care instructions
- Signature.

Because these areas are relevant to veterinary surgical procedures, they may be considered for inclusion in the veterinary operative report.

Since none of these fields are required in the veterinary profession, each practice and/or teaching institution must decide which are most applicable to their needs.

From the selected fields, surgical templates can be devised. These templates can be tailored to the procedure and include a series of fill-in-the-blank statements to facilitate data entry.

In human medicine, templates have been shown to improve compliance with standards for documentation.(2, 17, 18) Data entry is more apt to be complete because the fill-in-the-blank statements jog the surgeon's memory so that s/he is less likely to omit key facts.

For example, as a surgeon relying on my own memory, I may forget to include the suture material and size in the operative report. However, if I were to rely upon a template, the following fill-in-the-blank statements would prompt me:

- Suture material _____
- Suture size _____

The fill-in-the-blanks format of most templates also prevents errors that stem from the "copy-and-paste" approach to medical documentation.

As veterinary students, it is tempting to select, copy, and paste the surgical report from Patient A to the file of Patient B, who has undergone the same surgical procedure. The act is well-intentioned: the documenter uses "copy-and-paste" with the intention to borrow identical data so as to save time.(19)

Unfortunately, in an attempt to make haste, deletions are often incomplete and Patient A-specific data remains in Patient B's file. This creates a paperwork trail that is inaccurate.

A different suture material or suture size may have been used for Patient B. This may seem like a minor detail; however, what if Patient B subsequently developed a suture reaction? If Patient B's operative report suffers from "cut-and-paste" syndrome, and contains the suture information from Patient A, then Patient B may be linked to an adverse outcome with Suture A, when in fact Suture B was the problem.

Templates can be customized for any surgical procedure and are an effective way of reducing this error: the skeleton provides a framework on which to build a patient-specific entry.

11.2 Client-Centered Written Communication: Discharge Statements

Healthcare is like a team sport: each member of the team has a contribution, without which, quality care is sacrificed. Just as a baseball team needs its shortstop, the healthcare industry relies upon the client to adhere to medical recommendations.

In veterinary medicine, outpatient compliance is dependent upon the client's ability to recall, understand, and follow through with instructions.

We know from the human medical literature that noncompliance is a huge barrier to healthcare. Despite recommendations from their providers, up to 40% of human medical patients do not comply.(20–27) This percentage climbs to 70% if major lifestyle changes are required, particularly those involving diet or exercise.(28–32)

Compliance is also a significant barrier to veterinary care. For example, consider the use of flea, tick, and heartworm preventatives. Despite recommendations from the veterinary team that clients initiate and maintain prophylaxis year-round, only approximately 50% of dogs owned in the U.S. receive heartworm prevention monthly.(33, 34)

Communication plays an important role in follow-up. In human healthcare, it has been shown that patients are 30% less likely to be readmitted to the hospital for the same problem for which they initially presented if they understand their physician's instructions: when to take medications and when to be rechecked.(35–37)

Understanding is a bridge to compliance and results in improved outcomes, increased patient satisfaction, and decreased treatment times.(38–40)

Memory also contributes to compliance or the lack thereof. Human patients forget anywhere from 40–80% of what was shared during a medical consultation, as soon as the visit concludes.(41) Of the information that is recalled, half may be remembered incorrectly.(42)

There is also an inverse relationship between the amount of information presented and the amount of information that is recalled.(41) The more information that is presented, the less that is remembered.(43)

Discharge statements evolved as a way to supplement the information that is recalled by clients, and to reinforce key concepts.(44) Human hospitals are required to provide discharge statements by the Centers for Medicare and Medicaid Services (CMS) and the Joint Commission on Accreditation of Healthcare Organizations (JCAHO).(44)

Veterinary hospitals are not universally required to do the same. U.S. veterinary hospitals that are accredited by the American Animal Hospital Association (AAHA) must provide discharge instructions(45). However, those without AAHA accreditation may or may not incorporate discharge statements into practice-specific protocols to facilitate discharge planning.

Similarly, veterinary clients in the U.K. are dependent upon their veterinarians to provide what they feel is necessary to successfully manage patient care at home, in accordance with the *Code of Professional Conduct* by the Royal College of Veterinary Surgeons (RCVS).(46)

Furthermore, just because a discharge statement is provided does not mean that it will be effective. Historically, printed materials from human emergency room discharges have demonstrated poor rates of comprehension.(47–49) Simply put, just because a discharge statement exists does not mean that it will be understood.

An effective discharge statement is a reference tool for caregivers. To be successful as a reference tool, it must be written for the appropriate audience, in this case, the veterinary client.

A discharge statement that is appropriate for its audience has the following features:

- It is easy to follow
- It is patient-specific.

Discharge statements that are easy to follow are direct and to the point. They do not lose the reader's interest by going off on tangents. They stick to the main path and focus on the big picture:

- What is wrong with the patient?
- How is the patient going to be treated?
- For how long is the patient going to be treated?
- How will we know that the patient is better?

Consider the hypothetical case of a canine patient that was diagnosed with urolithiasis on a Saturday afternoon and is scheduled to undergo cystotomy two days later.

The patient's discharge statement reads:

DIAGNOSIS: Bladder stones

Bladder stones are concretions of one or more minerals. The most common stones that form are struvite or oxalate, but there are also cystine and urate stones. Certain breeds are predisposed to each type. Certain diets also predispose the patient to each type. Other predisposing factors include urinary pH (if the pH is too low or too high), and whether or not the patient has previously had a urinary tract infection.(50)

Bladder stones arise when the minerals that compose them precipitate in the urine as crystals. Initially, these crystals are microscopic: they may appear on a urinalysis. Eventually, these crystals accumulate like specks of sand. More and more crystals form around these specks until they become big enough to be seen on an X-ray. At a certain point, they become so large that they may become lodged in the urinary tract, causing an obstruction. Some stones are able to be dissolved rather than surgically removed, but that takes time. It also may increase the risk of obstruction as smaller stones start travelling down the urethra. We also don't know which type of stone is inside the bladder right now, so we would have to guess – and we could guess wrong.(50)

We have therefore decided to take Danby to surgery on Monday morning to surgically remove the stones. Please do not give Danby anything to eat after 11 p.m. on Sunday night. It is okay for Danby to drink water. Please arrive by 7:30 a.m. on Monday morning so that we can prepare Danby for the procedure.

Although the information contained above is relevant to the case and provides the client with a solid overview of urolithiasis, it runs the risk of providing too much information. There are so many facts clumped together that the reader may get lost before s/he finds what is important:

- When to withhold food
- Whether it is okay to offer water
- When to deliver Danby to the clinic on Monday morning.

It would be in the patient's best interest to provide an abbreviated discharge statement with the key points, and a separate client education handout on urolithiasis.

The abbreviated discharge statement could include the following:

DIAGNOSIS: Bladder stones

To prevent these from lodging within Danby's urinary tract, we have elected to remove the stones surgically on Monday morning.

In preparation for surgery, please do not feed Danby after 11 p.m. on Sunday night. It is okay for Danby to drink water. Please arrive by 7:30 a.m. on Monday morning so that we can prepare Danby for the procedure.

Please refer to "Bladder Stone" handout in the event that you wish to learn more about Danby's condition.

This document is much more concise. The reader is easily able to pick out the information that is most relevant to the patient and is more likely to follow through because the instructions were easy to find.

Understand that the attention span of the average adult is fleeting.(51) When lectured to, attention maxes out at 10–15 minutes.(51, 52) When we engage in everyday activities, attention span is even further reduced: it is on the order of seconds.(52)

Consider these facts when writing discharge statements for our clients.

Clients are, by nature, easily distracted. This tendency is only magnified when we ask them to weed through extraneous material. If we bury the key concepts in fluffy monologues, is it any wonder that our instructions are rarely followed?

To improve the odds that our instructions are heard, recalled, and followed, we ought to limit discharge statements to what is essential. In addition, we should lead with the most important information, the one take-away that you really need the client to recall. Contrary to popular belief, what is read first is more often remembered than what is read last.(51, 52)

Discharge statements must also contain easily understood language. Remember the purpose of the discharge statement, and for whom it was written. Medical jargon should be eliminated or, at the very least, defined. The discharge statement should unite the client and veterinarian in case management rather than divide them because of language.

Speak at the client's level, rather than expect the client to meet you at yours. This is challenging because every client is different and you are expected to adapt to each, not always knowing his/her level of comprehension.

In general, consider that health literacy is poor. In the U.S., 20% of adults read at or below a fifth grade level.(53) However, most healthcare resources are written at twice the difficulty of that level.(53)

Simplifying language compensates for poor health literacy. It also makes it less likely that a client feels talked down to or unable to ask a clarifying question for fear of seeming ignorant.

For example, consider writing:

- *Upset stomach* instead of *dyspepsia*
- *Bloody stool* instead of *hematochezia*
- *Straining to urinate* instead of *stranguria*
- *Low potassium* instead of *hypokalemia.*

Note that there is a difference between writing simply and using "baby talk." Although some clients may appreciate "baby talk," it is best to avoid certain words and phrases until you know your clients better.

For example, it sounds more professional to write, "upset stomach," than "upset tummy."

Keeping in mind the need to simplify the discharge statement, consider breaking it into sections or main ideas.

Below is one approach to segmenting the discharge statement into bite-sized, manageable chunks that are easy for the client to reference:

- Diagnoses
- Prognosis
- Case summary
- Feeding instructions
- Exercise restrictions (if applicable)

- Medications
- Additional care required
- What to watch for
- When to recheck.

Refer to Figure 11.1 for a sample discharge statement that makes use of this approach.

Referencing Figure 11.1, consider that the word, *diagnoses*, refers to the patient's problem list. This includes problems for which the patient presented, active problems, problems without a definitive diagnosis, and historical, but relevant, problems.

As an example, let us review the case of a 6-year-old Boxer dog that presented on emergency for ingestion of a chicken carcass. The dog was admitted for monitoring. It ultimately digested the carcass without endoscopic or surgical retrieval. However, during diagnostic imaging, urolithiasis was diagnosed.

Under *diagnoses* for this patient, you may include:

- Indigestion
- Bladder stones.

You may also include qualifiers such as "active" or "ongoing," "resolved" or "resolving."
For example:

- Indigestion – *resolved*
- Bladder stones – *active*.

Other qualifiers may include "cause unknown" or "under investigation."

Referencing Figure 11.1, consider that *medications* refer to newly prescribed drugs as well as ones that the patient may already be taking.

Medications that are listed should include the following information in one easy-to-spot location:

- Medication name
- Dose
- Route of administration
- Frequency of administration
- Special instructions for storage and/or administration

PATIENT DISCHARGE FORM

Patient Identification Number: _____

Patient Name: _____

Client Name: _____

Thank you for bringing _____ to _____ [Insert Name of Veterinary Clinic]

      DIAGNOSES:

      PROGNOSIS:

      CASE SUMMARY:

      TEST RESULTS:

      TESTS PENDING:

    FEEDING INSTRUCTIONS:

    EXERCISE RESTRICTIONS:

      MEDICATIONS:

     **ADDITIONAL CARE
      REQUIRED:**

    WHAT TO WATCH FOR:

     WHEN TO RECHECK:

Discharged by:_____

I have read and understand the above instructions.

Client's Signature:_____

Veterinarian's Signature: _____

Veterinarian's Name: _____

Clinic Name: _____

Clinic Address:_____

Clinic Contact Information: _____

Figure 11.1 Sample template for patient discharge statement

- Potential adverse effects
- How long the patient is anticipated to be taking the medication
- How many tablets or milliliters are being sent home with the patient
- Number of refills.

Use capitalized, bolded, or underlined words to emphasize instructions, such as:

- START
- CONTINUE
- DISCONTINUE
- DISCONTINUE IF YOU NOTICE _____
- INCREASE DOSE from _____ to _____
- DECREASE DOSE from _____ to _____
- INCREASE DOSING FREQUENCY from _____ to _____
- DECREASE DOSING FREQUENCY from _____ to _____
- RECHECK BEFORE STOPPING MEDICATION
- RECHECK AFTER STOPPING MEDICATION
- GIVE _____ MINUTES BEFORE _____
- GIVE _____ MINUTES AFTER _____
- REFRIGERATE
- SHAKE WELL
- DO NOT CRUSH
- DO NOT GIVE WITH CHEESE.

In addition, tailor the discharge statement to the patient.

Generic statements are less likely to have impact because they may not seem relevant to this patient's care.

Be specific about how the diagnosis or the treatment recommendations may affect *this* patient.

Instead of writing, "This medication may cause vomiting in dogs," consider the alternative:

- "This medication may cause Fluffy to vomit."

11.3 Veterinarian-Centered Written Communication: Referral Letters

As the profession of veterinary medicine has expanded to include specialty practice and emergency/critical care services, it is becoming more common for veterinary patients to have a network of care providers rather than a single full-service clinician.(54)

Although generalists have the ability to manage a broad spectrum of medical and surgical cases, there may come a time when a procedure or treatment is beyond the scope of their expertise. When this occurs, veterinarians in the U.S. and in the U.K. are bound by the American Veterinary Medical Association (AVMA) and the Royal College of Veterinary Surgeons (RCVS) respectively to arrange for the continued care and treatment of the patient.(55)

There are over 11,000 U.S.-based and 3,300 European-based veterinary specialists in over 20 distinct disciplines.(56, 57)

In the U.S., generalists may seek out the expertise of diplomates of the American Board of Veterinary Practitioners (ABVP) or the AVMA American Board of Veterinary Specialties (ABVS).(56, 58)

In the U.K., veterinary surgeons may seek out colleagues who have secured Certificates in Advanced Veterinary Practice (CertAVP) or board specialization via the European Board of Veterinary Specialisation.(57, 59)

In addition to referral for specialty care, patients may be referred out of necessity for: (55, 60, 61)

- Emergency coverage
- 24-hour in-patient monitoring
- Second opinion/inconclusive diagnosis
- Assessment of decompensating medical condition
- Managing client dissatisfaction with the attending clinician.

In order to make a referral, the burden falls upon generalists to become familiar with the range of services that are available within the vicinity of the area in which they practice.

Recommendations for referral should be geographically sound, with consideration given to the time-sensitive nature of the patient's specific needs.(60)

Subsequent communication with the client and receiving veterinarian is paramount to the successful transfer of care.

Although the details of oral communication with both parties are beyond the scope of this text, anticipated outcomes of referral should be communicated openly so that expectations can be clarified. The more individuals that are involved in caring for a patient, the more opportunities there are for miscommunication or misperceptions to arise.

Maintaining an open dialogue prior to and at the time of referral sets the stage for coordinated continuity of care.

However, oral communication alone is insufficient. AAHA forums were held in six U.S. cities between November 2006 and April 2007. These forums confirmed that written communication enhances a team-based approach to patient care.(54)

Most specialists prefer that referrals include a written case summary that either accompanies the patient or, ideally, arrives at the specialty center in advance of the appointment.(54)

The majority of specialty practices have templates available online to guide the referring veterinarian to provide the information that will be most helpful to the specialist.

Refer to Figure 11.2 for a sample template.

PATIENT REFERRAL FORM

Date: _____

Referring Veterinarian's Name: _____

Referring Veterinarian's Clinic: _____

Phone Number: _____ Fax Number: _____

Email: _____

Preferred Contact Method: ❑ Phone ❑ Fax ❑ Email

REFERRED TO:	❑ Behavior ❑ Dermatology ❑ Internal Medicine ❑ Neurology
	❑ Cardiology ❑ Imaging ❑ Ophthalmology ❑ Surgery
CHIEF COMPLAINT:	
RELEVANT HISTORY	
PHYSICAL EXAM FINDINGS	
DIAGNOSTIC TESTS	❑ Bloodwork ❑ Imaging ❑ Histopathology ❑ Other: _____ _____ _____ Please attach copies of results
TENTATIVE DIAGNOSIS/ RULE-OUTS	
TREATMENT / MEDICATIONS	
ANTICIPATED OUTCOME	

Figure 11.2 Sample template for referring veterinarian to complete for the benefit of the receiving veterinarian

Although a universal template would benefit the generalist, the reality is that each specialty requires different sets of patient data. Creating a form that suits everyone's needs would be challenging because even specialists within the same discipline have different information preferences and needs.

Therefore, whenever considering referral of a patient, direct your web browser to the specialty practice's home page to see if referral forms have been provided. If so, complete the requested form prior to or at the time of the appointment.

Specialists have historically expressed frustration that very few referring veterinarians follow through with providing the case history that is so desired.(54)

If the referral form does not provide the space to do so, you should still provide a case summary for the receiving veterinarian.(54) A case summary is specific to the referring problem, and can either take the form of a typed letter detailing relevant case history or a copy of the relevant SOAP note(s).

Typed is preferred to handwritten so that the information provided by the referring veterinarian is legible.(54, 62)

Recall the journalist's approach to history-taking that was covered in Chapter 4, and rely upon the five Ws to construct your case summary: (63, 64)

- Who?
- What?
- When?
- Where?
- Why?

For example, consider a 5-year-old, castrated male, Labrador Retriever that is being referred to the oncologist to stage lymphoma:

- Who?

    - this question is answered by the patient's signalment

- What?

    - this question is answered by the referred problem: the patient presented to the generalist for acute onset of bilateral firm swellings
    - when these swellings were aspirated, cytologic evaluation demonstrated findings that were consistent with lymphoma

- When?

    - this question is answered by tracking the timeline of events: the patient presented to the generalist yesterday
    - for three days prior to presentation at the generalist's, the patient was quiet, depressed, and inappetent

- Where?

  - this question is answered by identifying the location: the bilateral firm swellings are palpable under the angle of the mandible

- Why?

  - this question is asking why the patient is being referred
  - this question is answered by outlining the client's expectations for case management: the client is seeking the oncologist's recommendations for systemic chemotherapy
  - in addition, the client would like information regarding potential adverse effects of chemotherapy, and for how long the patient is likely to be in remission.

Note that a case summary is *not* a Xeroxed, scanned, or faxed copy of the patient's entire life history.(54) Full medical records are often too lengthy to be of use: data that is relevant to the referred problem has a tendency to be buried under items that are unrelated to the presenting complaint.

For example, an orthopedic surgeon who will be consulting with the owner of a 10-year-old dog with bilateral ruptured cranial cruciate ligaments (RCCL) does not need ten years' worth of data that discusses how the patient had roundworms as a puppy and a urinary tract infection at 2 years old.

On the other hand, the orthopedic surgeon *does* need to know that the left pelvic limb suffered from RCCL six months ago and that the patient was prescribed:

- A high fiber, weight loss diet
- Non-steroidal anti-inflammatory medications
- Opioids
- Over-the-counter glucosamine-chondroitin.

The orthopedic surgeon *does* need to know that the patient responded well to therapy until last week, when it became acutely lame on the right pelvic limb after chasing a Frisbee. RCCL on the right pelvic limb was diagnosed by palpation at that time. Radiographic exam was recommended but declined; the client anticipated having radiographs taken by the specialist.

Instead of faxing over the complete medical record, provide a complete history of the referred problem.(54) Include only those records that are relevant or may be relevant to the consultation.(54)

As a second example, consider a 12-year-old cocker spaniel that has no medical issues other than a new murmur that requires referral to a cardiologist for an echocardiogram. The cardiologist will benefit from a case summary that includes when the murmur was first identified, how (if at all) the murmur has progressed, whether or not the patient has clinical signs related to the murmur, any recent comprehensive laboratory work, and a list of any current medications. The rest is extraneous information that will not benefit the cardiologist's evaluation of the patient. If anything, having access to 12 years' worth of information may obstruct the process.

However, medical cases are not always that straightforward. When dealing with neurological complaints, particularly those that present atypically or over an extended period, it may be challenging to pinpoint precisely when the problem began. The clinical signs for which the patient presented three weeks ago may or may not be related to today's referred problem. There is a gray zone. When in doubt, include this material in the case summary or ask the veterinarian whom you will be referring to, to outline his/her preference.

In addition to providing a history that is specific to the referred problem, your case summary should include relevant data in the form of: (54, 61, 62)

- Laboratory tests: bloodwork, urinalysis, fecal analysis, etc.
- Electrocardiograms (ECGs)
- Imaging reports
- Histopathology reports.

Diagnostic data is especially relevant to case management. When diagnostic information is excluded from case summaries, the specialist is forced to either repeat diagnostic testing or make recommendations for case management without access to the whole picture. Neither situation is fair to the receiving veterinarian, the client, or the patient.

To be considerate of all parties involved in the referral process, the referring veterinarian needs to provide timely, accurate, and concise yet complete documentation. Doing so sets the stage for the professional and coordinated transfer of patient care from one provider to another. High-quality documentation facilitates high-quality referral.

11.4 Electronic Correspondence

The digital age has added a new layer to the veterinarian–client relationship: the potential for electronic correspondence. Many veterinary clients are accustomed to communicating in this manner with their human healthcare team; it is not uncommon for them to transfer those expectations onto the veterinary community.(65)

Email is efficient and timely.(66, 67) Many clients appreciate that they can initiate conversation without a telephone call and at any hour of the day or night, when something is on their mind.(65)

Veterinarians may in turn appreciate that they can receive an update instantaneously, without having to play phone tag, and that they can respond at their convenience, in between other tasks, without risking a phone call that may derail their appointment schedule.

Veterinarians may also find themselves working into the night and worry that a phone call after hours may not be well received because it is too late. An email seems like an easy solution: unlike a telephone call, it does not run the risk of waking up a client.(65)

When electronic correspondence is appropriate, it can facilitate patient care and follow-up. However, electronic correspondence also walks a thin line at times, between what is medically warranted and what is abusive.(66, 68)

Email may be misused or overused by clients. It is all too easy to send an inquiry (or two! or three!) with the click of a button and expect an instantaneous answer. Clients may forget that veterinarians are not always "on."

Veterinarians should not be expected to return messages around the clock, particularly when they are off duty.

Yet because an email can be sent 24-7, clients may be unreasonable in their expectations for a rapid turnaround time. Clients may send an email and expect to hear back right away. If they do not, they may become frustrated or disillusioned with the system, not understanding that their expectations were unrealistic.

Clients may also take advantage of the hiding behind a computer screen to express their discontent with veterinary care. It is often easier to speak freely when there are no checks and balances, as in a face-to-face conversation. For some, email is a good way to blow off steam. This is a concern for the veterinary profession as a whole because this represents a breach of email etiquette. Clients that use email in this manner are crossing the line and need to be called out.

An additional concern regarding electronic correspondence is that individuals who are not clients, but are family, friends, or coworkers, or otherwise connected to, clients, may reach out for medical advice. These individuals may have expectations that a "curbside consultation" is appropriate. They may expect free advice or even a diagnosis without submitting to a consultation.

It is neither professionally nor legally sound to dispense medical advice to these individuals because no veterinarian–client–patient relationship (VCPR) exists.

In order to navigate these situations and reduce the likelihood that they will arise, private practices and teaching institutions need to establish an email policy with clear-cut boundaries that address email etiquette.

The veterinary team needs to be clear and consistent in terms of what types of questions will be answered, the acceptable turnaround time for a response, who will be responsible for the response, and how that correspondence will be recorded in the medical record.(67)

For example, clinics may elect to set the following ground rules: (65)

* No "urgent" matters are to be discussed via email. All emergency situations need to be handled either via telephone or in person during office hours
* All queries that ask for a diagnosis will be advised to schedule an appointment
* No immediate response should be expected. On average, expect a response to take 24–48 hours.

In addition to establishing ground rules that match their own comfort level, private practices and teaching institutions are responsible for ensuring that their policies do not breach professional or legal standards.

For example, in the absence of a VCPR, practices may need to establish a standard response to unsolicited emails from those with whom no such relationship exists:(69)

> It is against the law for our practice to dispense veterinary medical advice without having a pre-established veterinarian–client–patient relationship. We would appreciate the opportunity to serve you. If you wish to make an appointment, please contact our practice at [insert telephone number].(69)

Individual veterinarians should also have the right to determine their own comfort level concerning electronic correspondence. For instance, veterinarians may elect to be selective about whom is granted access to their professional email account.(65)

Veterinarians also need to protect themselves by keeping business and pleasure separate, as is standard operating procedure for human medical doctors.(67) Work-related and personal correspondence should never cross paths.(67)

Veterinarians should maintain separate accounts: one for business and one for private communications.(67) Joint accounts blur the boundaries of what is and is not professionally appropriate. Furthermore, employers may legally have the right to review any correspondence that is associated with their system.(70)

Email may be an increasingly common form of communication in healthcare, but be cautious. Understand that it may lead to or worsen miscommunication.(66, 68) Unlike face-to-face conversation, which has the added benefit of facial expression, body language, eye contact, and tone of voice, email lacks non-verbal cues that assist with message interpretation.(67) It is easy to misconstrue words or assume that comments were intended a certain way, particularly if the subject matter is controversial or emotionally intense.(67, 71)

For example, the following phrases may be well intentioned; however, your client may read between the lines and come up with a different conclusion:

- "You should . . ."
- "The problem is . . ."

- "As I mentioned before . . ."
- "I know how you feel . . ."

"You should" may come across as being sincere and respectful in person, particularly when you, the veterinarian, have been asked to provide advice.

However, in writing, "you should" may strike the reader as being blunt, condescending, or dismissive. "You should . . ." could be replaced with "I recommend that . . ." The latter comes across in writing as being softer and gentler.

Likewise, "the problem is . . ." sounds harsh. People also don't tend to like to hear that there is a problem. It sends hackles up the back. It also makes it sound like a brick wall that is insurmountable.

Instead of creating this image in the reader's mind, lead with: "The challenging aspect of managing Lucifer's diabetes is that he does not prefer to eat set meals; however, one solution to work around his feeding habits would be to . . ."

Although this acknowledges there is a concern, it also provides the reader with a strategy for how to best address it.

"As I mentioned before . . ." may have been intended to jog the reader's memory, but it may come across that you do not appreciate having to repeat yourself.

"I know how you feel . . ." may be an honest attempt at empathy. However, do we ever *truly* know what it is like to be another person? We may try to put ourselves in their shoes, but no matter how hard we try, we can never be them.

A client in grief does not want to hear that you know how s/he feels. The truth is that *no one* does.

Emotionally charged emails are particularly difficult to navigate because they often invoke negativity in the reader. For example, if a veterinarian is the recipient of an angry email, it may be tempting to react defensively or passive-aggressively. The knee-jerk reaction is often to reply immediately and hit send before taking the time to process what was read and what you've said.

In these circumstances, it is best not to respond via email. There is too much room for miscommunication. Emotions act as accelerants: they fuel the fire. When an emotional situation arises, it is imperative that electronic correspondence be taken out of the equation and instead handled the old-fashioned way: face-to-face.

Thinking before hitting "send" is always a good rule of thumb. Review your words and consider the following:

- Is what I am typing clear?
- Is there a way to make my words even more clear?
- Is there any likelihood that what I wrote could be misconstrued?
- What can I do to decrease the chance that what I wrote could be misunderstood?
- Would I be comfortable if this email was inadvertently sent to a family member?
- Would I be comfortable if this email was inadvertently sent to my boss?
- Would I be comfortable if this email was inadvertently made public?
- Am I confident that my words are professional?
- Am I confident that my words are the best reflection of who I am as a veterinarian?

If there ever is any doubt that what you are writing could be misinterpreted or could be damaging either to your character or to the integrity of your practice, stop before you hit "reply."

Once you hit "send," you cannot take back your words. They are not private. They become a permanent record.(67)

It has been said that you should "be conservative in what you send and liberal in what you receive."(72) Nowhere is this more true than in electronic correspondence. After all, email provides a false sense of security: its contents are not confidential.(67) Your words can come back to haunt you.

So be cautious. Be alert. Be aware of what you write and how you write it. Carry yourself in your writing as a professional. Be courteous always, and most importantly, be safe.

END-OF-CHAPTER SUMMARY

The SOAP note is not the only form of documentation in veterinary medicine. In addition, a patient's medical record may include:

- Operative reports
- Discharge statements
- Referral letters
- Email correspondence.

Just as there are no universal guidelines for the structuring of SOAP notes in veterinary medicine, there are no universal guidelines for these types of records. Their structure and format vary widely between veterinarians and from practice to practice. There is no one "right" approach.

Veterinarians, veterinary team members, and veterinary students must adopt a method that works best for them and that can be consistently reproduced.

Operative reports typically include the following:

- Date/time/name of procedure
- Description of incision: i.e. size, location
- Description of procedure
- Complications during procedure(s)
- Description of closure: i.e. suture material, suture size
- Antibiotic prophylaxis (where applicable)
- Postoperative care instructions
- Signature.

Templates for operative reports reduce errors of omission.

Discharge statements should be:

- Written for the client
- Easy to follow
- Patient-specific.

Referral letters should include a case summary that is complete with regards to the presenting complaint and relevant in terms of both case history and diagnostics.

Each practice should set boundaries regarding electronic correspondence with clients.

References

1. Wilson JF. Law and Ethics of the Veterinary Profession. Yardley, PA: Priority Press, Ltd.; 2000.

2. Laflamme MR, Dexter PR, Graham MF, Hui SL, McDonald CJ. Efficiency, comprehensiveness and cost-effectiveness when comparing dictation and electronic templates for operative reports. AMIA Annu Symp Proc. 2005:425–429.

3. Hossain T, Hossain N. Guidance of writing general surgical operation notes: a review of the literature. International Surgery Journal. 2015;2(3):326–330.

4. Mathew J, Baylis C, Saklani AP, Al-Dabbagh AR. Quality of operative notes in a district general hospital: a time for change? Internet J Surg. 2003;5:116–119.

5. Latimer K, Pendleton C, Martinez A, Subramanian PS, Quinones-Hinojosa A. Insight into glaucoma treatment in the early 1900s: Harvey Cushing's 1905 operation. Arch Ophthalmol. 2012;130(4):510–513.

6. Comprehensive Accreditation Manual for Hospitals: The Official Handbook: Joint Commission on Accreditation of Healthcare Organizations; 2004.

7. Good Surgical Practice England: Royal College of Surgeons of England; 2014. Available from: file:///C:/Users/renglar/Downloads/GSP%202014%20web.pdf

8. Lefter LP, Walker SR, Dewhurst F, Turner RW. An audit of operative notes: facts and ways to improve. ANZ J Surg. 2008;78(9):800–802.

9. Novitsky YW, Sing RF, Kercher KW, Griffo ML, Matthews BD, Heniford BT. Prospective, blinded evaluation of accuracy of operative reports dictated by surgical residents. Am Surg. 2005;71(8):627–631; discussion 31–32.

10. Flynn MB, Allen DA. The operative note as billing documentation: a preliminary report. Am Surg. 2004;70(7):570–574; discussion 4–5.

11. Zaninelli M, Campagnoli A, Reyes M, Rojas V. The O3-Vet project: integration of a standard nomenclature of clinical terms in a veterinary electronic medical record for veterinary hospitals. Comput Methods Programs Biomed. 2012;108(2):760–772.

12. State of the Industry Report: 2016 Highlights. North American Pet Health Insurance Association; 2016.

13. Tange HJ, Hasman A, de Vries Robbe PF, Schouten HC. Medical narratives in electronic medical records. Int J Med Inform. 1997;46(1):7–29.

14. Dunn L. Small animal practice: billing, third-party payment options, and pet health insurance. Vet Clin North Am Small Anim Pract. 2006;36(2):411–418, vii.

15. Veterinary Practice Partners (VPP). Pet Insurance: Still No Breakthrough in the US Market. VETPulse. 2013;4(Fall). Available from: http://www.vetpartners.com/wp-content/uploads/2016/05/VETPulse-Volume-4-Fall-2013.pdf.

16. General Standards: American Animal Hospital Association; 2017. Available from: https://www.aaha.org/professional/membership/general_standards.aspx

17. Henry SB, Douglas K, Galzagorry G, Lahey A, Holzemer WL. A template-based approach to support utilization of clinical practice guidelines within an electronic health record. J Am Med Inform Assoc. 1998;5(3):237–244.

18. Crist-Grundman D, Douglas K, Kern V, Gregory J, Switzer V. Evaluating the impact of structured text and templates in ambulatory nursing. Proc Annu Symp Comput Appl Med Care. 1995:712–716.

19. Hirschtick RE. A piece of my mind. Copy-and-paste. J Am Med Assoc. 2006;295(20):2335–2336.

20. Martin LR, Williams SL, Haskard KB, Dimatteo MR. The challenge of patient adherence. Ther Clin Risk Manag. 2005;1(3):189–199.

21. DiMatteo MR. Enhancing patient adherence to medical recommendations. J Am Med Assoc. 1994; 271(1):79, 83.

22. DiMatteo MR. Social support and patient adherence to medical treatment: a meta-analysis. Health Psychol. 2004;23(2):207–218.

23. DiMatteo MR. Evidence-based strategies to foster adherence and improve patient outcomes. JAAPA. 2004;17(11):18–21.

24. DiMatteo MR. Variations in patients' adherence to medical recommendations: a quantitative review of 50 years of research. Med Care. 2004;42(3):200–209.

25. DiMatteo MR, DiNicola DD. Achieving Patient Compliance: The Psychology of the Medical Practitioner's Role. New York: Pergamon Press; 1982. xvi, 335 pp.

26. Martin KA, Bowen DJ, Dunbar-Jacob J, Perri MG. Who will adhere? Key issues in the study and prediction of adherence in randomized controlled trials. Control Clin Trials. 2000;21(5):195s–199s.

27. Laederach-Hofmann K, Bunzel B. Noncompliance in organ transplant recipients: a literature review. Gen Hosp Psychiat. 2000;22(6):412–424.

28. Dishman RK. Compliance/adherence in health-related exercise. Health Psychol. 1982;1:237–267.

29. Dishman RK. The measurement conundrum in exercise adherence research. Med Sci Sport Exer. 1994;26(11):1382–1390.

30. Brownell KD, Cohen LR. Adherence to dietary regimens. Behav Med. 1995;20:149–154.

31. Katz DL, Brunner RL, St Jeor ST, Scott B, Jekel JF, Brownell KD. Dietary fat consumption in a cohort of American adults, 1985–1991: covariates, secular trends, and compliance with guidelines. Am J Health Promot. 1998;12(6):382–390.

32. Chesney MA. Factors affecting adherence to antiretroviral therapy. Clin Infect Dis. 2000;30 Suppl 2:S171–176.

33. Gates MC, Nolan TJ. Factors influencing heartworm, flea, and tick preventative use in patients presenting to a veterinary teaching hospital. Prev Vet Med. 2010;93(2–3):193–200.

34. Cummings J, Vickers L, Marbaugh J, editors. Evaluation of veterinary dispensing records to measure "clinic compliance" with recommended heartworm prevention programs. Heartworm Symposium; 1995. American Heartworm Society.

35. Parker C, Griffith DH. Reducing hospital readmissions of postoperative patients with the martin postoperative discharge screening tool. J Nurs Adm. 2013;43(4):184–186.

36. Novak CJ, Hastanan S, Moradi M, Terry DF. Reducing unnecessary hospital readmissions: the pharmacist's role in care transitions. Consult Pharm. 2012;27(3):174–179.

37. Senior Care Guidelines Task Force, Epstein M, Kuehn NF, Landsberg G, Lascelles BD, Marks SL, et al. AAHA senior care guidelines for dogs and cats. J Am Anim Hosp Assoc. 2005;41(2):81–91.

38. Marcus C. Strategies for improving the quality of verbal patient and family education: a review of the literature and creation of the EDUCATE model. Health Psychol Behav Med. 2014;2(1):482–495.

39. Behar-Horenstein LS, Guin P, Gamble K, Hurlock G, Leclear E, Philipose M, et al. Improving patient care through patient–family education programs. Hospital Topics. 2005; 83(1):21–27.

40. Advancing Effective Communication, Cultural Competence, and Patient- and Family-Centered Care: A Roadmap for Hospital. Oakbrook Terrace, IL: The Joint Commission; 2010.

41. Kessels RP. Patients' memory for medical information. J R Soc Med. 2003;96(5):219–222.

42. Anderson JL, Dodman S, Kopelman M, Fleming A. Patient information recall in a rheumatology clinic. Rheumatol Rehabil. 1979;18(1):18–22.

43. McGuire LC. Remembering what the doctor said: organization and adults' memory for medical information. Exp Aging Res. 1996;22(4):403–428.

44. Zeng-Treitler Q, Kim H, Hunter M. Improving patient comprehension and recall of discharge instructions by supplementing free texts with pictographs. AMIA Annu Symp Proc. 2008:849–853.

45. Principles of Veterinary Medical Ethics of the AVMA: American Veterinary Medical Association; [5/30/17]. Available from: https://www.avma.org/kb/policies/pages/principles-of-veterinary-medical-ethics-of-the-avma.aspx

46. Royal College of Veterinary Surgeons. Code of Professional Conduct for Veterinary Surgeons. 2018. Available from: https://www.rcvs.org.uk/setting-standards/advice-and-guidance/code-of-professional-conduct-for-veterinary-surgeons/.

47. McCarthy DM, Engel KG, Buckley BA, Forth VE, Schmidt MJ, Adams JG, et al. Emergency department discharge instructions: lessons learned through developing new patient education materials. Emerg Med Int. 2012;2012:306859.

48. Zavala S, Shaffer C. Do patients understand discharge instructions? J Emerg Nurs. 2011; 37(2):138–140.

49. Engel KG, Heisler M, Smith DM, Robinson CH, Forman JH, Ubel PA. Patient comprehension of emergency department care and instructions: are patients aware of when they do not understand? Ann Emerg Med. 2009;53(4):454–461 e15.

50. Ettinger SJ, Feldman EC, Côté E. Textbook of Veterinary Internal Medicine: Diseases of the Dog and the Cat. 8th ed. St. Louis, MO: Elsevier; 2017.

51. Khan S. Why Long Lectures Are Ineffective. TIME; 2012. Available from: http://ideas.time.com/2012/10/02/why-lectures-are-ineffective/.

52. Middendorf J, Kallish A. The "Change-Up" in Lectures. The National Teaching and Learning Forum [Internet]; 1996:1–12. Available from: https://docstull.files.wordpress.com/2013/11/the-generalist-integration.pdf

53. What Is Health Literacy? Center for Health Strategies; 2008. Available from: http://www.chcs.org/media/What_is_Health_Literacy.pdf

54. Donnelly AL. Focus on Referral Issues. Trends magazine [Internet]; 2007: November/December. Available from: https://www.aaha.org/public_documents/professional/resources/focusonreferral.pdf

55. VCPR: The Veterinarian-Client-Patient Relationship: American Veterinary Medical Association; 2017. Available from: https://www.avma.org/KB/Resources/Reference/Pages/VCPR.aspx

56. AVMA American Board of Veterinary Specialties: American Veterinary Medical Association; 2017. Available from: https://www.avma.org/ProfessionalDevelopment/Education/Specialties/Pages/default.aspx

57. European Board of Veterinary Specialisation: EBVS; 2017. Available from: http://ebvs.eu/

58. The Standard of Excellence in Veterinary Care: American Board of Veterinary Practitioners; 2017. Available from: http://abvp.com/

59. Royal College of Veterinary Surgeons: Certificate in Advanced Veterinary Practice (CertAVP); 2017. Available from: http://www.rcvs.org.uk/education/lifelong-learning-for-veterinary-surgeons/certificate-in-advanced-veterinary-practice-certavp/

60. AAHA Referral and Consultation Guidelines; 2013: November. Available from: https://www.aaha.org/public_documents/professional/guidelines/aahareferralguidelines2013.pdf

61. Guidelines for Equine Veterinary Case Referral; 2013. Available from: https://aaep.org/sites/default/files/Guidelines/Guidelines%20for%20Equine%20Veterinary%20Case%20Referral_final_11112013.pdf

62. Referrals and Second Opinions: Royal College of Veterinary Surgeons; 2016. Available from: https://www.rcvs.org.uk/advice-and-guidance/code-of-professional-conduct-for-veterinary-surgeons/supporting-guidance/referrals-and-second-opinions/

63. Journalistic Writing: Eastern Washington University; 2016. Available from: http://research.ewu.edu/c.php?g=403887

64. Arnold C, Cook T, Koyama D, Angeli E, Paiz JM. How to Write a Lead: Purdue University; 2013. Available from: https://owl.english.purdue.edu/owl/resource/735/05/

65. Kay N. Communicating with Your Vet: Email Etiquette. The Bark [Internet]; 2011. Available from: http://thebark.com/content/communicating-your-vet

66. O'Brien JA. Netiquette: e-mail for group practices. J Med Pract Manage. 2007;22(4):201–203.

67. Albersheim S. E-mail communication in paediatrics: ethical and clinical considerations. Paediatr Child Health. 2010;15(3):163–168.

68. Purcell TJ. Enhancing electronic communications between team members by establishing best practices: a communications specialist's perspective. Drug Inf J. 2001;35(1):35–40.

69. DeVille K, Fitzpatrick J. Ready or not, here it comes: the legal, ethical, and clinical implications of E-mail communications. Semin Pediatr Surg. 2000;9(1):24–34.

70. Ceresia P, Crolla DA. Using Email Communication with Your Patients: Legal Risks. Ottawa: Canadian Medical Protective Association; 2009.

71. Saul JM. E-mail etiquette: when and how to communicate electronically. Cause/Effect. 1996;2:50–251.

72. Hambridge S. Netiquette Guidelines. Intel Corporation; 1995. Available from: http://www.ietf.org/rfc/rfc1855.txt

Chapter 12

An Introduction to Scientific Writing

The focus of this text, through Chapter 11, has been to introduce the concepts of medical writing. For veterinary professionals who actively practice medicine, medical writing constitutes an essential component of day-to-day clinic life. Without proper documentation through medical writing, patient care and continuity of care cannot be maximized. Veterinarian–client communication and veterinarian–veterinary team communication will fall short, and the details of case management are likely to get lost in translation. At its core, medical writing exists to protect the tripartite relationship in the veterinary medical profession: the veterinarian, the client, and the patient. Without competent medical writing, this relationship falls apart.

Scientific writing fosters a different relationship. The purpose of scientific writing is to disseminate clinical observations in order to:(1)

- Share knowledge about clinical presentation of disease
- Determine risk or patient predisposing factors for developing disease
- Share knowledge of new, proposed, or amended treatments of disease
- Demonstrate how new approaches to case management may alter disease progression
- Document adverse or unexpected effects of treatment
- Evaluate the effectiveness of different treatment modalities
- Identify new areas of research that will facilitate case management.

Scientific writing is the means by which the profession of veterinary medicine advances.

Veterinary medicine is anything but a static field. The profession evolves because the scientific community works tirelessly to address deficits in our knowledge base. These efforts are often published in the form of:(1)

- Case reports, to document unique conditions or novel approaches to treatment
- Editorials, to stimulate debate and encourage critical thinking within the profession
- Conference abstracts, to summarize data and share preliminary results
- Review articles, to track knowledge on a given subject
- Full-length manuscripts, to publish the results of studies that were specifically designed around research questions.

The byproducts of research vary broadly in terms of topic, length, format, and audience.

Studies also exhibit great diversity in terms of approach. Some reflect quantitative research methods, based on benchtop laboratory analysis with hard numbers. Quantitative research also tends to answer the questions: "what?", "which?", "when?", and "how often?"(2–4)

For example, a quantitative study may seek to answer the following research questions:

- "What is the impact of drug 'x' on hepatocellular enzymes?"
- "Which drug induces the most rapid remission for Stage 3a lymphoma?"
- "When does neutropenia occur following chemotherapy using drug 'y'?"
- "How often do surgical complications occur following routine ovariohysterectomy by new graduates?"

Others take on a qualitative approach to document observations, behaviors, and motivations through interviews and focus groups.(2, 5–7) This approach is frequently used by psychologists, who often ask the questions, "why?" and "how?"

Veterinary science must also ask "why?" and "how?" because ultimately it is a people-driven profession. The veterinarian cannot treat the patient without interacting with the client. Therefore, how veterinarians communicate to clients and why clients react the way they do matters to the profession. These types of questions are just as important from a research perspective as questions about what drug "x" does to disease "y."

Quantitative and qualitative research are not exclusionary. They often lean on or lead to one another.(2, 8) For example, in market research, a quantitative study may first evaluate how many people purchased the topical flea product, "z," from their primary care veterinarian. A follow-up qualitative study may then seek to determine how effectively these consumers perceived whether the product met expectations.

The ultimate goal of research, irrespective of the method used, is to produce high-quality, reproducible, evidence-based medicine.(1) Research that promotes critical thinking and new approaches to case management is in demand, particularly in the areas of public health, pathology, infectious disease, and translational medicine.(9–14)

Early student exposure to comparative and translational medicine is valuable. If students are shown how veterinary practitioners can influence interdisciplinary efforts, they can begin to see themselves as a necessary link between the advancement of animal and human health.(9–14)

The concept of "One Health" emerged during the 21st century to symbolize collaboration among the health professions.(9) However, veterinary medicine has long contributed to biomedical research and comparative medicine.(15)

For example:

- In the late 1800s, Daniel Salmon studied infectious diseases and how quarantines could contain their spread(16)
- In 1898, Loeffler and Frosch discovered that foot-and-mouth disease was caused by a virus(17)

- In 1908, Ellerman and Bang demonstrated the role of viruses in leukemia(18)
- In 1933, Richard Shope discovered that rabbit papillomatosis was caused by a virus(19)
- In 1973, Eklund and Hadlow identified that scrapie was caused by prions.(20)

Advancements in veterinary medicine continue to be made because of ongoing research.

As medicine evolves and the need for research grows, veterinarians can draw upon their unique position at the interface between animal and human disease. Just as practitioners can contribute to medicine, so, too, can they contribute to research.

In order to participate in research and publish, the veterinary profession must be exposed to and gain familiarity with scientific writing.

Scientific writing is not often taught by veterinary educators but is essential to master so that observations and knowledge can be more readily shared. Here, scientific writing is *introduced* so that you know what types of opportunities exist and how best to pursue them.

12.1 Deciding Where to Publish

Students may only be exposed to a handful of journals throughout the veterinary curriculum; however, there are over 250 veterinary journals worldwide.(1) Each journal has its own scope, that is, its breadth and depth of content as well as a particular audience of subscribers.

Some journals may provide broad-based coverage of the veterinary profession, for instance, the *Journal of Veterinary Internal Medicine*. Others, such as *Veterinary Pathology*, may limit themselves to a particular specialty area.

Understanding for whom each journal is written and what the journal focuses on is the first step towards assessing whether or not your material will be an appropriate fit. A short summary of the journal, its audience, and its aim is usually visible on the homepage of the journal.

For example, consider the *Journal of Veterinary Medical Education* (JVME):

> As an internationally distributed journal, JVME provides a forum for the exchange of ideas, research, and discoveries about veterinary medical education.(21)

From this description, it is evident that JVME is intended for distribution to veterinary medical educators.

Alternatively, consider the *Journal of the American Veterinary Medical Association* (JAVMA):

> Published twice monthly, this peer-reviewed, general scientific journal provides reports of clinical research, feature articles and regular columns of interest to veterinarians in private and public practice.(22)

The reader will understand that JAVMA is intended for distribution to practicing veterinarians.

Once the audience of the journal is clear, explore the content of the journal. Browse a recent issue. Alternatively, a table of contents should be easily accessible online. For example, the homepage for JVME, http://jvme.utpjournals.press/loi/jvme, allows one to navigate the table of contents for both the in-print and upcoming issue.

Navigating the table of contents allows one to see how the journal is arranged.

For example, Volume 44, Number 2 of JVME outlines topics according to the following subject headers: (21)

- Letters to the Editor
- Animal Welfare and Animal–Human Interaction
- Student Attainment and Wellbeing
- Communication and Interpersonal Skills
- Assessment and Interpretation
- Clinical Education.

Note that this outline may vary from issue to issue, so it behooves the reader to examine several recent issues to appreciate the variety. An assessment of the content helps the reader to ascertain the kinds of topics that are considered newsworthy.

If what is currently in print is in line with the content that you are interested in publishing, the next step is to examine the journal's manuscript instructions for authors. Within this section, each journal outlines the categories for which authors are allowed to submit.

For example, as of June 2017, the categories for which JAVMA was accepting submissions included: (23)

- Views
  - Letters to the Editor
  - Commentaries
  - Viewpoint Articles
- Scientific Reports
  - Original Studies
  - Clinical Reports
  - Review Articles.

Each category then provides journal-specific guidelines for manuscript preparation. These guidelines include the manuscript's format and organization.

Formatting guidelines are detailed and include:

- Page size
- Margins
- Font
- Font size
- Spacing
- Alignment of text
- Line numbering.

The manuscript's organization will depend very much upon the type of submission and the journal.

For example, an Original Study in JAVMA must be structured as follows: (23)

- Title page
- Structured abstract
  - Objective
  - Design
  - Animals (or sample)
  - Procedures
  - Results
  - Conclusions and Clinical Relevance
- Text
- Acknowledgments
- Footnotes
- References
- Figures
- Tables.

Each journal has its own specific requirements to which authors must adhere.

You can see now why it is so important to select a journal *before* writing the manuscript. The format that is considered appropriate for one journal may not be suitable for another.

12.2 Additional Characteristics of Journals to Consider

Another important consideration when selecting where to display your work is the quality of journal. Not all journals offer the same amount of visibility, prestige, and impact factor.

12.2.1 Visibility

Visibility refers to the audience, that is, who will be able to access the journal. Prior to the internet, journals were available in print only. Visibility was thus subscription-based. The individual or the organization, for example, an academic library, purchased subscriptions. In some cases, membership fees for professional organizations paid for the journal. Non-subscribers could still purchase individual journal issues; however, the cost to do so was – and still is – substantial.

Because the reader covers the cost of publication, authors of publications in subscription-based journals are not responsible for footing the bill. In print, subscription-based journals have a budget. This budget determines how many pages can be produced per issue to manage costs. Therefore, print journals have to be selective about which articles appear in which issues.(24)

The internet changed the world's access to science. Many journals transitioned from being available in print only to being available online. Visibility has increased as selectivity has decreased: online journals no longer have to worry about page budget, the production cost per page per issue. This has led to an explosion of publications in science.(24)

As the number of publications in science grows, the audience for them continues to widen. Open-access journals provide free access to all articles online, meaning that anyone can access any article of interest.(1, 25)

"Golden road" open-access journals are most common: although readers are not required to pay for access, authors are required to fund publication. Employers or grants can cover the cost; however, the fees can be quite substantial.(1)

When dealing with "golden road" open-access journals, it is important to understand what is being paid for, and to consider the kind of product in which your work will be showcased.

Many open-access journals provide editorial support along with high-quality peer review.(1) These journals maintain high standards and refuse to sacrifice quality of content for quantity.(24)

12.2.2 The Concept of "Predatory Journals"

Not all open-access journals are reputable. These so-called "predatory journals" provide the illusion of high-quality publication, but lack the infrastructure to support legitimate peer review.(1, 24, 26–29) They may also disguise unqualified individuals as scientific experts on editorial boards.(1)

The incentive for "predatory journals" is purely financial. Each publication provides a steady stream of revenue for the publisher regardless of whether or not the manuscript is scientific and high quality.(24) A complicating factor is that the resultant articles are often indexed within such reference tools as Google Scholar, making it increasingly difficult to discern science from pseudoscience.(24)

Lists of questionable open-access journals are available online from a variety of sources.(30, 31)

"Beall's List" is a well-known blacklist within the academic community, compiled by a University of Colorado librarian.(32) Although controversial, "Beall's List" succeeds at shedding light on a very real phenomenon in academic publishing.

In order to not fall victim to a scam, it is critical that authors of manuscripts discern the reputation of a journal.(1) Quality work belongs in a quality resource.

When in doubt, conduct an extensive review of the journal and publisher. Search for recognizable identifiers. A reputable journal should provide the name and credentials of the editor and the editorial board. "Predatory journals" tend not to identify key staff or provide proof of academic expertise.(24, 33)

"Predatory journals" also tend not to disclose the whereabouts of their publishing headquarters. They may link themselves in title to a particular region of the world, without any actual ties to the geographical zone. For instance, a journal that contains

"Canadian" in its title but lacks any physical ties to the country should raise a red flag. (24, 33)

"Predatory journals" are rarely lone fish in the sea. They often exist as part of a series by "predatory publishers." These promote scores of journals, each one broad-based, in an attempt to cover every topic and every medical specialty.(24, 33)

"Predatory publishers" are effective spammers. Be wary of form letter solicitations, particularly those that ask for manuscripts for topics outside of or on the periphery of your area of expertise.(24, 33)

Finally, compare journal content to standards that have been established by the Open Access Scholarly Publishers Association (OASPA) and the Committee on Publication Ethics (COPE).(33)

12.2.3 Prestige

Prestige refers to the "it" factor. In every field, there are journals that are considered the "go to" or the "gold standard" resource. These journals have built an elite reputation from producing substantial, high caliber work and maintaining that level of high quality over an extended period. These journals are overseen by strong editorial boards and rigorous peer-review processes that select for the best, most current, most relevant, and most scientific manuscripts.(1)

Consult your mentors and known experts in the field to determine which journals carry this reputation.(1)

Consider asking your professors, attending clinicians, and colleagues, "If you only had time to reference three journals in veterinary medicine, which would they be?" The answers that you are given will help to separate the elite resources, those with solid reputations, from the rest of the pack.

12.2.4 Impact Factor

The impact factor is one aspect of journal metrics, the attempt to rank scientific journals within like fields.(1) Specifically, impact factors measure how often an article in journal "x" is cited during a specific time interval. Many impact factors are based upon two years; some are based upon five years.

Let's consider a two-year impact factor for Journal "x" in the year 2012.

The impact factor is equal to:

[The number of citations in 2012 to articles published in 2010–2011 in Journal "x"] divided by [The number of articles published in 2010–2011]

This numerical value allows for comparison between journals within the same discipline, which are likely to share a similar audience with similar scientific needs or pursuits. The higher the numerical score, the higher the ranking within a given discipline.

All known impact factors are published by Thomson-Reuters annually in Journal Citation Reports (JCR).(1)

For example, in 2015, the following human medical journals received the following impact factor scores: (34)

- *New England Journal of Medicine*: 59.558
- *The Lancet*: 44.002
- *Journal of the American Medical Association*: 37.684
- *The Lancet Oncology*: 26.509
- *The Lancet Neurology*: 23.468.

Compare these to 2015 impact scores for the following veterinary medical journals: (34)

- *Veterinary Record*: 1.741
- *Journal of the American Veterinary Medical Association*: 1.501
- *Journal of Feline Medicine and Surgery*: 1.211
- *American Journal of Veterinary Research*: 1.124
- *Journal of Veterinary Medical Education*: 0.901.

It would be inappropriate to compare the impact score for the *Veterinary Record* with the impact score for the *New England Journal of Medicine* because their audiences are very different. Such a comparison would be akin to evaluating apples against oranges.

Note that impact factors are one of many factors to consider when deciding where to publish. Impact factors were never intended to be used as stand-alone data. They are, at best, imperfect measurements.

They can be fabricated by "predatory publishers," who may post them hoping that a novice researcher will not confirm their accuracy. They can also be manipulated if journals promote self-citation.

However, impact factors provide a starting point for the quantitative evaluation of journal quality.

They help you to gauge your chances of being published within a given journal. Journals with lower impact factors are more likely to consider manuscripts from unknown authors, whereas journals with higher impact factors are more prestigious and may publish only those who are considered the field's leading experts.(25)

END-OF-CHAPTER SUMMARY

Scientific writing is an important means by which the profession of veterinary medicine disseminates information about clinical observations.

Scientific writing includes:

- Case reports
- Editorials
- Conference abstracts
- Review articles
- Full-length manuscripts.

Deciding what to publish requires the author to consider where to publish.

Each journal is written for a specific audience and has certain areas of emphasis in terms of what it chooses to print.

For example, the *Journal of Veterinary Medical Education* (JVME) is a forum for veterinary educators to exchange ideas about curricular advancements. JVME is not in the habit of publishing case reports to evaluate novel dosing of drug "y" for the medical management of disease "x."

It is critical to determine where your topic has the best "fit." Understanding for whom each journal is written and the journal's area of interest is the first step towards assessing the "fit."

The second step is to examine the journal's instructions for authors. Each journal outlines open categories for submission. Each category then provides journal-specific guidelines for manuscript preparation. These guidelines include the manuscript's format and organization, and they must be adhered to if the manuscript is even to be considered for publication.

In addition, the author should consider the following journal-specific factors:

- Visibility
- Prestige
- Impact factor.

Beware of so-called "predatory journals." These may appear to offer opportunities for high-quality publication. However, they lack:

- Quality control
- Expert leadership
- Legitimate peer review.

References

1. Christopher M, Young K. Writing for Publication in Veterinary Medicine: A Practical Guide for Researchers and Clinicians; 2015. Available from: http://www.wiley.com/legacy/wiley blackwell/gmspdfs/VETWritingforPub/pubData/source/VETWritingforPubPDF.pdf

2. Creswell JW. Qualitative Inquiry & Research Design: Choosing Among Five Approaches. 2nd ed. Thousand Oaks, CA: Sage Publications; 2007. xvii, 395 pp.

3. Hoy WK. Quantitative Research in Education: A Primer. Los Angeles: SAGE; 2010. xvi, 141 pp.

4. Martin WE, Bridgmon KD. Quantitative and Statistical Research Methods: From Hypothesis To Results. 1st ed. San Francisco: Jossey-Bass; 2012. xviii, 476 pp.

5. Horvat EM, Heron ML. The Beginner's Guide to Doing Qualitative Research: How to Get into the Field, Collect Data, and Write up Your Project. New York: Teachers College Press; 2013. xvi, 160 pp.

6. Merriam SB, Tisdell EJ. Qualitative Research: A Guide to Design and Implementation. 4th ed. San Francisco, CA: Jossey-Bass; 2016. xix, 346 pp.

7. Maxwell JA. Qualitative Research Design: An Interactive Approach. 3rd ed. Thousand Oaks, CA.: SAGE Publications; 2013. xi, 218 pp.

8. Johnson B, Christensen LB. Educational Research: Quantitative, Qualitative, and Mixed Approaches. 4th ed. Thousand Oaks, CA.: SAGE Publications; 2012. xxvi, 621 pp.

9. Rosol TJ, Moore RM, Saville WJ, Oglesbee MJ, Rush LJ, Mathes LE, et al. The need for veterinarians in biomedical research. J Vet Med Educ. 2009;36(1):70–75.

10. Hubbell JA, Richardson RC, Heider LE. Workforce needs for clinical specialists at colleges and schools of veterinary medicine in North America. J Am Vet Med Assoc. 2006; 229(10):1580–1583.

11. Hoblet KN, Maccabe AT, Heider LE. Veterinarians in population health and public practice: meeting critical national needs. J Vet Med Educ. 2003;30(3):287–294.

12. Cardiff RD, Ward JM, Barthold SW. 'One medicine–one pathology': are veterinary and human pathology prepared? Lab Invest. 2008;88(1):18–26.

13. Critical Needs for Research in Veterinary Science: Reports Funded by National Institutes of Health. Washington, DC: National Academies Press; 2005.

14. National Need and Priorities for Veterinarians in Biomedical Research: Reports Funded by National Institutes of Health. Washington, DC: National Academies Press; 2004.

15. Tasker JB. Standing on the Shoulders of Giants: Foundations in Veterinary Medicine for the Advancement of Human Welfare. Tamarac, Florida: Llumina Press; 2008.

16. Cima G. LEGENDS: America's First DVM; 2013. Available from: https://www.avma.org/News/JAVMANews/Pages/130301m.aspx

17. Mahy BW. Introduction and history of foot-and-mouth disease virus. Curr Top Microbiol Immunol. 2005;288:1–8.

18. Syverton JT, Ross JD. The virus theory of leukemia. Am J Med. 1960;28:683–698.

19. Shope RE, Hurst EW. Infectious papillomatosis of rabbits: with a note on the histopathology. J Exp Med. 1933;58(5):607–624.

20. Kim K. The Social Construction of Disease: From Scrapie to Prion. Abingdon, Oxon; New York, NY: Routledge; 2007. xvii, 253 pp.

21. Journal Profile: AAVMC. Available from: http://jvme.utpjournals.press/loi/jvme

22. About JAVMA: American Veterinary Medical Association. Available from: https://www.avma.org/news/journals/pages/javma-about.aspx

23. JAVMA Instructions for Authors: Journal of the American Veterinary Medical Association. Available from: https://www.avma.org/News/Journals/Documents/javma-ifa.pdf
24. Beall J. Best practices for scholarly authors in the age of predatory journals. Ann R Coll Surg Engl. 2016;98(2):77–79.
25. Taylor RB. The Clinician's Guide to Medical Writing. New York: Springer; 2005. xiv, 266 pp.
26. Gasparyan AY, Yessirkepov M, Diyanova SN, Kitas GD. Publishing ethics and predatory practices: a dilemma for all stakeholders of science communication. J Korean Med Sci. 2015;30(8):1010–1016.
27. Shen C, Bjork BC. 'Predatory' open access: a longitudinal study of article volumes and market characteristics. BMC Med. 2015;13:230.
28. Shamseer L, Moher D, Maduekwe O, Turner L, Barbour V, Burch R, et al. Potential predatory and legitimate biomedical journals: can you tell the difference? A cross-sectional comparison. BMC Med. 2017;15(1):28.
29. Hansoti B, Langdorf MI, Murphy LS. Discriminating between legitimate and predatory open access journals: report from the International Federation for Emergency Medicine Research Committee. West J Emerg Med. 2016;17(5):497–507.
30. Sorokowski P, Kulczycki E, Sorokowska A, Pisanski K. Predatory journals recruit fake editor; 2017. Available from: http://www.nature.com/news/predatory-journals-recruit-fake-editor-1.21662
31. Kolata G. A Scholarly Sting Operation Shines a Light on 'Predatory' Journals. NY Times [Internet]; 2017. Available from: https://www.nytimes.com/2017/03/22/science/open-access-journals.html
32. Beall J. Beall's List of Predatory Journals and Publishers; 2016. Available from: http://beallslist.weebly.com/
33. Beall J. Criteria for Determining Predatory Open-Access Publishers; 2012. Available from: https://scholarlyoa.files.wordpress.com/2012/11/criteria-2012-2.pdf
34. Thomson-Reuters. Journal Citation Report 2015. Available from: file:///C:/Users/renglar/Downloads/2016%20journal%20citation%20reports%20(thomson%20reuters%202015)%20(1)%20(1).pdf

Chapter 13

Deciding What to Write

A successful manuscript is planned. It doesn't just happen.

Any manuscript can be written well, but if it is not grounded in good science, then it will not withstand the peer-review process.(1)

Planning requires an investment of time and self-reflection. You need to start by asking yourself the following questions:(2)

- What is the scope of my current work?
- What within the scope of my current work interests me?

Passion for the subject matter is critical. Passion is what fuels those long days and nights of research, writing, and revisions. Passion is what commits you to the process, regardless of the outcome, and drives you towards the finish line.

If you do not care about the topic, then why should others?

Yet passion alone is insufficient. Passion may lead you to conceive a project. However, if no one shares your passion or if the project's results are not applicable to colleagues in your field, then the project is not relevant to the current veterinary medical literature. The project must answer a clinical question, one that others need to care about.(2)

You must ask yourself if the selected topic interests others.

If your interests are timely and relevant to the work of others, you should proceed with the selected topic. Like an inverted pyramid, start broadly, then narrow the focus.

Refine your topic by asking the following questions:

- What within the scope of my topic has already been explored, and to what degree?
- What within the scope of my topic remains uncharted territory?

To answer these questions, you must conduct a literature review. A literature review is an important step in the planning process to establish whether your idea has already been conceptualized in print.(2)

There are a multitude of electronic databases for literature searching, including ones that are tailored for the medical and veterinary medical professions.(2) Consider

PubMed,(3) Medline via Raven,(4) Centre for Agriculture and Biosciences International (CABI),(5) Web of Science,(6) and the Cochrane Library.(7)

These databases are typically free of charge to conduct searches, and they provide links to abstracts of applicable articles. However, unless they are open access, you may require a subscription to access full-text articles.

It is also wise to consult a preferred search engine, such as Google Scholar,(8) particularly if the key words in your database search did not turn up much by way of content. Adapt your search. Test out synonyms as alternate key words. It is possible that your content area has been published before, just under a slightly different search than your original.

If prior work in your content area has been published, examine it closely. There may be an area or an angle that has yet to be explored.

In addition, consult the references at the end of each article to see if any sources overlap with your topic or could be of help in providing you with background information. Background information anchors your research by providing you with the current knowledge base. This material is what will round out your introduction, should you proceed with your research project and reach the manuscript-writing phase.

Prior endeavors to research your chosen topic may also provide you with clues as to how to develop your research question further and tips on study design. Perhaps researchers of a similar study acknowledged limitations to their design that you could correct for in a subsequent project.

Conducting a literature review is time-intensive. However, the results of such a thorough investigation are fruitful in that they facilitate your planning. They tell you what has been done before and why, as well as opportunity areas that have yet to be explored.

When you discover the opportunity area that is right for you, you need to ask yourself the following:

- Is it possible for you to study what has not been done before?
- Who, if anyone, do you need to partner with to facilitate this research?

Research is often a joint effort. Rarely is the primary investigator the sole researcher on any given project.

Do not be afraid to reach out to mentors both within and outside of the university setting. Invite others to the table to brainstorm, particularly if you are a novice. Learn from others' areas of expertise, and learn from others' mistakes.

The time you put into planning the project is well worth the investment. Planning allows you to troubleshoot potential glitches now as opposed to later, when a poorly executed study yields unreliable and unpublishable conclusions.(1)

The product of brainstorming is a well-developed research question. Research questions require creativity and critical thinking. It is not enough to replicate what has been printed in the literature before.

Consider, for example, the following questions:

- How effectively does butorphanol provide analgesia following onychectomy?
- How does thrombin contribute to the coagulation cascade?
- How does phenobarbital increase hepatic enzymes?
- What are the adverse effects of heparin?

These questions run the gamut from basic physiology to pharmacology, and are appropriate for veterinary students to ask in order that they understand the process or the drug that may be at work.

These questions form the basis of learning issues that students may be responsible for researching and reporting back to the house officers on the clinic floor.

However, these questions are not new. These questions have been asked before. These questions have answers. Those answers just have to be found.

An effective research question pushes beyond existing knowledge to ask what is still yet to be discovered. In this respect, research questions require thinking outside of the box to postulate a hypothesis that is testable, using a design study that is reproducible.

Study design is beyond the scope of this text and requires forethought. However, you should consider the following well in advance of proceeding with the collection of research data: (1)

- What, if any, animals do you need to conduct this research?

    - how many do you need?
    - can this number be justified?
    - are there non-animal alternatives?
    - what is the source of the animals?
    - are animals naturally diseased or experimental models of disease?

        - not all journals accept research that involves experimentally induced disease, for example the *Journal of Small Animal Practice*(1)

    - who is responsible for approving animal use?

        - in the U.S., the Institutional Animal Care and Use Committee (IACUC) oversees the use of animals in research at the level of the institution. At the national level, the Animal Welfare Act (AWA) regulates animal research, and is enforced by the U.S. Department of Agriculture (USDA)(9)
        - in the U.K., the Animal Welfare and Ethical Review Body (AWERB) regulates animal use in research at the local level; at the national level, animal research must be approved by the Home Office by way of the Animals in Science Committee(10)

- What, if any, human subjects do you require to conduct this research?

    - how many subjects do you need?
    - can this number be justified?
    - who is responsible for approving the use of human subjects?

- in the U.S., the Institutional Review Board (IRB) is responsible for providing approval and oversight so as to minimize risks to subjects, protect vulnerable populations, and ensure the provision of informed consent(11)
- in the U.K., peer review of research involving human subjects is required by the U.K. Research Integrity Office (RIO) in order to preserve ethical boundaries and protect patient confidentiality(12)

- What, if any, equipment do you need to conduct this research?
- What, if any, funds do you need to secure to facilitate this research?
- What, if any, approvals and authorizations do you need to gather to proceed?

In addition to these background considerations, study design must consider the following: (13)

- Which type of study is being pursued?

  - is the study retrospective or prospective?
  - is the study case-controlled or cross-sectional?
  - is the study intended to be a clinical trial, and if so, is it randomized or controlled?
  - is the study intended to be a systematic review or a meta-analysis?

- What variables will be studied?
- What is/are the control(s)?
- What outcomes will be analyzed?
- How will outcomes be analyzed?
- Is sample size adequate for the planned statistical analysis?
- What are potential obstacles to the collection of data?
- How will these obstacles be overcome?
- What, if any, obstacles are insurmountable?
- How will you ensure that these insurmountable obstacles do not prevent the results from being valid?

Consulting someone with experience in research, particularly in your area of expertise and with experience conducting research using your study design of choice, is necessary. Research mentors provide essential guidance and can assist with troubleshooting before fatal flaws in study design occur.(1)

In addition, consulting research reporting guidelines before collecting study data can serve as a quality control to make sure that what you produce is accurate and unbiased. Consider, for example, Reporting Guidelines for Randomized Controlled Trials for Livestock and Food Safety (REFLECT).(14) REFLECT provides a 22-item checklist to facilitate the reporting of outcomes pertaining to livestock health, production, and food safety.(14)

Note that research-reporting guidelines are scant in veterinary medicine, and few have been adopted formally by veterinary journals. However, human medical research reporting guidelines can be valuable tools to round out your approach to the methods section and how you intend to capture results. In fact, REFLECT was the product of a steering committee's efforts to adapt the human creation, CONSORT, to veterinary medical trials.(14) CONSORT, STARD, ARRIVE, STROBE, and PRISMA are just a few of the human-grade medical reporting guidelines that can be examined prior to study design to improve the quality of the end result.(1)

Understand that research is a process. Your work evolves as you grow as a researcher. What you initially conceived of and what you initially set out to do may transform into a very different research aim, one that is stronger and more original.

It is the evolution of research that makes it so exciting. Yet the same factors that make research dynamic and enticing can also make it daunting. At times it may seem impossible to begin when there is so much pre-work to consider.

Recognize that the pre-work is an important first step. Planning study design is a critical part of completing a manuscript. Think of the planning process as a precursor for authorship, in which:

* Your literature search translates into what will become your manuscript's introduction
* Your study design translates into what will become your materials and methods
* Your collected data translates into your results and discussion.

What you put into planning becomes the shape of the manuscript that you will write. Your efforts in advance will pave the way for a stronger finish line.

END-OF-CHAPTER SUMMARY

Original research articles are a common type of scientific manuscript in all healthcare professions, including veterinary medicine.

Writing an original research article requires planning.

You start by asking yourself the following questions:

* What is the scope of my current work?
* What within the scope of my current work interests me?

Once you have selected a topic that overlaps with your area of expertise and professional interests, you need to refine it by asking yourself the following questions:

* What within the scope of my topic has already been explored, and to what degree?
* What within the scope of my topic remains uncharted territory?

A literature search is required to answer these questions. Several databases have been tailored to meet the needs of healthcare professionals, including:

- PubMed
- Centre for Agriculture and Biosciences International (CABI)
- Web of Science.

These databases sift through their collections based upon key words that you have listed in your query.

The result of any query is a list of links to abstracts. Unless the article is open-access, many full-text versions require journal subscriptions in order for you to obtain a copy.

Full-text articles are an important starting point for you to explore your area of interest in depth.

The references that are listed at the end of full-text articles can be equally valuable in that they help to expand your search of what has already been explored and what remains to be discovered.

Seek out mentors to encourage your journey through scientific writing. You may also need to consider partnering with one or more colleagues in order to facilitate your research.

Brainstorming and study design are important next steps. Pre-work is worth the investment of time and energy. It helps you to troubleshoot before problems arise.

References

1. Christopher M, Young K. Writing for Publication in Veterinary Medicine: A Practical Guide for Researchers and Clinicians; 2015. Available from: http://www.wiley.com/legacy/wiley blackwell/gmspdfs/VETWritingforPub/pubData/source/VETWritingforPubPDF.pdf
2. Taylor RB. The Clinician's Guide to Medical Writing. New York: Springer; 2005. xiv, 266 pp.
3. PubMed. Bethesda, Maryland: National Center for Biotechnology Information, U.S. National Library of Medicine. Available from: https://www.ncbi.nlm.nih.gov/pubmed?otool=igbcambulib
4. Medline via Raven: University of Cambridge. Available from: http://www.lib.cam.ac.uk/eresources/fulllist.php?search=%25&search_term=medline+%28ovid%29&type=%25&submit=Find+resources
5. CABI VetMed Resource. Available from: http://www.cabi.org/vetmedresource.
6. Web of Science 2017. Available from: http://apps.webofknowledge.com/WOS_GeneralSearch_input.do?product=WOS&search_mode=GeneralSearch&SID=2BzsPZF5FCYySgLgvDW&preferencesSaved
7. Cochrane Library. Available from: http://www.cochranelibrary.com/
8. Google. Available from: https://scholar.google.com/
9. National Research Council (U.S.). Science, Medicine, and Animals: A Circle of Discovery. Washington, DC: National Academies Press; 2004. 52 pp.

10. Speaking of Research. Available from: https://speakingofresearch.com/facts/animal-research-regulations-in-the-uk/

11. Information on Protection of Human Subjects in Research Funded or Regulated by U.S. Government: U.S. Department of Health and Human Services. Available from: https://www.hhs.gov/1946inoculationstudy/protection.html

12. Research Involving Human Participants, Human Material or Personal Data: UK Research Integrity Office. Available from: http://ukrio.org/publications/code-of-practice-for-research/3-0-standards-for-organisations-and-researchers/3-7-research-involving-human-participants-human-material-or-personal-data/

13. Literature Reviews: Types of Clinical Study Designs: Georgia State University. Available from: http://research.library.gsu.edu/c.php?g=115595&p=755213

14. O'Connor AM, Sargeant JM, Gardner IA, Dickson JS, Torrence ME, Consensus Meeting Participants, et al. The REFLECT statement: methods and processes of creating reporting guidelines for randomized controlled trials for livestock and food safety by modifying the CONSORT statement. Zoonoses Public Health. 2010;57(2):95–104.

Chapter 14

Writing the Original Research Article

Recall from Chapter 12 that each journal provides its own set of guidelines for what constitutes an appropriate submission. As such, always consult the journal of interest for formatting requirements. What one journal considers standard may not be in line with another journal's expectations.

That being said, original research articles typically follow the structure that is outlined below:(1)

- Introduction
- Methods
- Results
- Discussion.

This format is recalled by the acronym IMRaD.(1, 2) IMRaD is an effective template to organize the structure of an original research article.

The title, key words, and abstract tack onto the beginning of IMRaD, whereas references, tables, and figures tack onto the end.

Note that although research articles follow this order in print, authors do not necessarily write these sections sequentially.(1) Many authors, for instance, write the abstract last.

Each author must decide how to approach manuscript writing in a way that is most logical for organizing his/her thoughts. Below is one example of staging the manuscript in a way that flows logically for this author.

14.1 Titling the Original Research Article

The author finds it easiest to start with the title to ground the project. Keep in mind that the first title is a draft that is likely to undergo revision as the manuscript evolves.

Consider, for example, the following title revisions by this author, in chronological order, from original to published title:

- "Using Standardized Clients to Discuss Animal Cruelty."
- "Using Standardized Clients to Practice Discussions about Animal Cruelty Reporting."
- "Using a Standardized Client Encounter to Practice Veterinary Team Discussions about Animal Cruelty Reporting."

- "Using a Standardized Client Encounter in the Veterinary Curriculum to Practice Veterinarian–Employer Discussions about Animal Cruelty Reporting."

The final title serves as the best reflection of the content in the body of the manuscript: it gained study-specific detail as the manuscript evolved.

In addition, titles should be concise and accurately report the intent of the study. Consider, for example, the following titles:

- "The effect of platelet-rich plasma on osseous healing in dogs undergoing high tibial osteotomy."(3)
- "The effect of acepromazine alone or in combination with methadone, morphine, or tramadol on sedation and selected cardiopulmonary variables in sheep."(4)
- "Effect of feed restriction and initial body weight on growth performance, body composition, and hormones in male pigs immunized against gonadotropin-releasing factor."(5)

Alternatively, titles may be informative; that is, they reflect the conclusion of the study:

- "Propofol protects against opioid-induced hyperresponsiveness of airway smooth muscle in a horse model of target-controlled infusion anesthesia."(6)
- "Lysine supplementation is not effective for the prevention or treatment of feline herpesvirus 1 infection in cats: a systematic review."(7)
- "High levels of acetoacetate and glucose increase expression of cytokines in bovine hepatocytes, through activation of the NF-κB signalling pathway."(8)

Titles usually also reference the study design. Consider, for example, the following titles:

- "A qualitative study to explore communication skills in veterinary medical education."(9)
- "Evaluating dog and cat owner preferences for Calgary-Cambridge communication skills: results of a questionnaire survey."

14.2 Considering Key Words

After titling the project, the author turns his/her attention to the key words. Key words or phrases augment the title and represent what readers are likely to search for so that databases can retrieve the article.(1) Some journals cap key words or phrases at a certain number. When there is no limit, most authors select four to eight.

Consider, for example, the article entitled, "Applicability of the Calgary-Cambridge Guide to Dog and Cat Owners for Teaching Veterinary Clinical Communications."(10) The key words and phrases that the authors selected were:

- Client perspective
- Communication skills
- Curriculum
- Focus group study
- Foundational and core communication skills
- Qualitative research
- Veterinary education.

Note that most of the key words and phrases are distinct from those found in the title. This is intentional. Key words and phrases are intended to supplement the title by allowing readers to find the article without knowing it by name. Readers rely upon indexes and search engines to catalogue materials by key word.

Consider an alternate example, "Differences in intestinal microbial metabolites in laying hens with high and low levels of repetitive feather-pecking behavior."(11)

The key words that the authors selected were:

- Laying hen
- Feather-pecking behavior
- Microbiota
- Biogenic amines
- Short chain fatty acids.

Neither biogenic amines nor short chain fatty acids appear in the title; however, if a reader were to search for these terms in a database, the article would be retrieved. Key words therefore facilitate an article's visibility.

14.3 The Introduction for the Original Research Article

The introduction follows the key words. Unless the manuscript is a review article, the purpose of the introduction is not to be comprehensive. In fact, many journals provide word limits for this section of the article. The purpose of the introduction is to grab the reader's attention. The introduction provides the "so what?" factor: this is what we know, this is what we need to know, and this is why it matters.(1)

Think of the introduction in the same way you would an inverted pyramid. Start with the big picture, then focus on key concepts as they relate to your study.

Consider, for example, a hypothetical research study about aortic thromboembolism (ATE) in cats. The structure and flow of the introduction for this study most logically starts with a broad-sweeping fact:

Aortic thromboembolism (ATE) is associated with hypertrophic cardiomyopathy in cats.(12–14)

The next few sentences of the introduction narrow the topic towards the research question:

> When it occurs, ATE carries a poor prognosis, particularly when clinical presentation involves multiple limbs.(14) Current medical management is largely supportive, and the client's decision to euthanize may depend upon whether pain management appears to be effective.(14) A new analgesic in human medicine demonstrates promise in the management of pain secondary to thrombus formation; however, its utility in cats has not been explored.

The introduction is further narrowed to the research question, hypothesis, and/or objectives:

> The authors hypothesized that drug "x" would more effectively manage feline pain secondary to ATE than the current standard of care, drug "y." Objectives were to 1) compare feline pain in patients with ATE that are managed with drug "x" to pain in patients managed with drug "y," 2) identify adverse events that occurred secondary to administration of drug "x," and 3) propose an effective dosing range for drug "x" in cats with ATE.

Finally, the introduction explains why the research question is relevant to the audience:

> If drug "x" more effectively and safely manages feline pain secondary to ATE as compared to drug "y," then owners may be more likely to treat ATE. If owners are more willing to treat ATE, then more cats may survive ATE to the point of discharge.

Headers may or may not be used to subdivide the introduction. This decision depends in large part upon the author's preference and the introduction's length. For example, let us reconsider the 2016 article by Englar et al.(10) This article made use of headers throughout the introduction in order to group similar topics:(10)

- "The impact of communication on human health care"
- "The development of communication skills as a clinical competency in human health care"
- "The impact of communication on veterinary health care"
- "The development of communication skills as a clinical competency in veterinary health care"
- "Developing a veterinary model of clinical communication."

Because this article introduced the role of communication in both human and veterinary health care, the use of headers was a logical way to structure the article to make it easier to follow.

14.4 Outlining the "Materials and Methods" Section in an Original Research Article

If the purpose of the introduction is to establish the research question, then the purpose of the "materials and methods" section is to explain how you answered the question. As such, the "materials and methods" section follows the introduction as a concise, yet complete, review of study design and statistical analysis.

The study design should be clear and draw from the hypothesis and objectives. The study design should paint a picture of the research that was conducted, when it was conducted, where it was conducted, and under whose authority and oversight.

Researchers should include all relevant details so that readers could recreate the experiment. However, the risk of full disclosure is that readers may get lost in the details, particularly if they are not experts in the content area.

Flow charts and other organizational diagrams can help to simplify complex study designs to keep readers engaged and to minimize confusion.

If the results of a pilot study influenced study design, then it is appropriate to include these. Otherwise, results do not belong in the "materials and methods" section.

In studies involving animal patients, the following details need to be recorded: (1)

- Source of animals
- Recruitment of animals
- Signalment of animals
- Housing of animals

    - group-housed vs. individually housed
    - randomized housing vs. grouping by characteristic, such as age or sex

- Other animal-related care
- Extent of research that was conducted

    - what was done to which groups of animals, with what frequency, over what period of time?
    - how were humane standards of animal research maintained?

- Were animals removed from the study? If so, why?

The procedure(s) must be detailed fully. Consider, for example, a study involving blood pressure. Concerning the measurement of blood pressure, the following details belong in the "materials and methods" section:

- Who measured blood pressure in the study?

    - one individual vs. multiple individuals
    - if multiple individuals were involved as measurers, then how were inter-measurer differences addressed in the study?

- What measurements of blood pressure were taken?

  - indirect or direct measurement
  - if indirect, were Doppler or oscillometric methods used?
  - if oscillometric methods were used, then what were the cuff size(s) and cuff location(s)?
  - brand name and manufacturer of all instruments used

- How often was blood pressure measured?

  - at what time points were measurements taken?

- How was blood pressure reported?

  - as a single value
  - as the average of a series of readings

- How was blood pressure recorded?

  - what units of measurement were ascribed to blood pressure?

- How were research subjects handled?

  - immediately before blood pressure measurements
  - in between blood pressure measurements
  - after blood pressure measurements.

Veterinary studies may also involve human subjects. For example, veterinary educators may evaluate the effect of training tool "y" on first-year veterinary students, or veterinarians may survey the public to identify key traits that are desirable in new graduates. When human subjects are involved, recruitment methods must be addressed, taking into consideration:

- Source of participants
- Inclusion criteria
- Exclusion criteria
- How are participants identified?
- How are participants recruited?
- Are there follow-up recruitment procedures?
- How are subjects enrolled?
- How can subjects remove themselves from the study?
- When can subjects remove themselves from the study?

In addition, the "materials and methods" section for research involving human subjects must outline the following ethical considerations: (15, 16)

- Were vulnerable populations recruited?

  - minorities
  - disabled

- pregnant
- institutionalized

- Were potential participants briefed on their rights as subjects?
- Were potential participants briefed on the anticipated benefits of the project?
- Were potential participants briefed on the anticipated risks of the project?
- Were participants compensated?
- Did participants provide informed consent?

After study design has been thoroughly reviewed, the "materials and methods" section should touch upon how statistical analysis was used to evaluate the study's results.(1) Specifically, readers need to be able to answer the following questions:

- Which statistical test(s) did the authors use to analyze the data?
- How was the level of statistical significance defined?

With regards to statistical testing, data analysis must be addressed for all quantitative and qualitative data. Quantitative data analysis may include: (17)

- Descriptive statistics

    - mean
    - median
    - inter-quartile range
    - standard deviation

- Specific tests

    - correlational tests
    - chi-square test
    - independent T-test
    - regression tests
    - non-parametric tests.

Qualitative data analysis may include: (18, 19)

- Content analysis
- Narrative analysis
- Thematic analysis.

A description of each method of data analysis is beyond the scope of this text.

Researchers should consult mentors in their content area during the planning phases of the project to establish which statistical test or set of tests best fits study design.

The goal is to pick one or more tests that most accurately analyze the project's results. In other words, the test should evaluate what you want to test. If the test does not achieve this function, then it is not an appropriate test for your study.

14.5 Results

If the purpose of the "materials and methods" section is to explain how you answered the research question, then the results section outlines the answers that were discovered along the way. As such, the results follow the "materials and methods" section and provide factual data methodically arranged for easy review.

The data that is pertinent, meaning that it relates back to the study's hypothesis and objectives, should be showcased.

Showcasing data is different than manipulating it to make it seem more impressive.

Data may be consolidated in figures or tables. These tools should be used selectively, when they provide value as stand-alone visual aids.(1)

Figures and tables should not be used just because they look aesthetically pleasing. If the contents can be summarized in text, then text is adequate and need not be replaced by a graphic design.

Follow the journal's guidelines for how to present figures and tables in the manuscript. Figures and tables may have specific requirements for being numbered, named, and captioned.

Journals may also have special requirements for color use, and often only allow color for online issues. Most figures and tables should therefore be adapted to grayscale on a background of white. Keys should be provided, as needed, to identify research groups, and fonts should be selected for readability rather than elaborateness.(1)

14.6 Discussion

If the purpose of the results section is to present the answers to the research question, then the purpose of the discussion is to provide an interpretation of those facts.

The discussion is not supposed to be a repeat of the results. The discussion should expand upon the results to make appropriate conclusions that can be linked back to the study's hypothesis and objectives.(1)

In addition, the discussion is an opportunity to acknowledge limitations in the study's design and consider future developments for research in the content area, knowing what we know now.(1)

Some, but not all, journals require a conclusion in addition to the discussion. Refer to the journal's guidelines to establish the content for this section.

14.7 The Abstract

The abstract is usually written last. It is also one of the most difficult to write because it must summarize the article's context and results within a limited word count.

Like the introduction, the abstract must draw the reader in, but with limited background information. The meat of the abstract is the study's rationale, design, results, and conclusion, all of which is typically stated in 350 words or less.(1)

If the abstract is the first section that the reader sees after the title, then why is it typically written last? To understand this concept, consider the alternative.

If the abstract is written first, then it runs the risk of being obsolete. Manuscripts evolve as they grow. They mature. Each draft represents a more refined version of the last. If the abstract is written before the manuscript undergoes revision, then the abstract will not match the tone, quality, content, or voice of the latest draft.

If the abstract does not reflect the tone, quality, content, or voice of the latest draft, then it inaccurately reflects the manuscript that follows. Because the abstract must function as a stand-alone synopsis of the manuscript, it must be precise, accurate, and consistent.

In the author's experience, the best way to achieve an up-to-date abstract is to draft it after the manuscript has found its voice and its purpose.

14.8 Revising the Original Research Article

Writing is a process. Rarely, if ever, is the first draft acceptable for publication.

Consider the first draft as a starting point, an opportunity to organize your thoughts into words on paper. However, the first draft often lacks precision and clarity. Preliminary thoughts and ideas are not necessarily coherent or articulate. Word choice may be off-kilter or inaccurate.

When you begin the revision process, ask yourself if the product is an accurate reflection of what you intended to say. Do the written words mean to others what they mean to you? Or is there room for error? Are there problem areas, assumptions, or misconceptions?

Read your draft aloud. Discover where you get tongue-tied. Identify run-on thoughts or awkward phrasing.

Consider transition statements: do sections flow logically, from one to the next?

Ask yourself if the terminology used throughout is accurate and consistent.

Most importantly, does it make sense to your audience?

All contributors to the manuscript should go through the process of self-review, critically assessing their work within the context of the manuscript as a whole. Only after collaboration in which all authors agree on a "final" draft should the circle of feedback widen to include those unrelated to the study.

Why is input from outside the study's circle of researchers so integral to the process of manuscript revisions? What we may think is clear, may be ambiguous to a colleague. It is therefore a good idea to ask for feedback from a colleague who lacks prior knowledge of the study. This colleague serves as an appropriate sounding board by sharing what is and is not clear, and which areas could benefit from clarification.

When seeking feedback, it is especially beneficial to ask someone with experience in scientific writing. A friend who is an exceptional poet may not be able to make head nor tail of an abstract.

Allow those who are experienced in the process to weigh in.

Be prepared for criticism and lots of red ink! Equate red ink with progress, rather than failure. Red ink means that the manuscript is salvageable; it just needs work.

Consider also leaning on mentors who are detail-oriented, grammatically correct editors. These individuals are helpful spot-checkers of spelling and grammar. These may seem like minor points of contention; however, first impressions count. Incorrect spelling and poor grammar can significantly detract from the presentation and the perceived quality and rigor of your manuscript.

Finally, consider asking for feedback from those with opposite writing styles to your own. If your writing tends to be long-winded or flowery, look to someone with a knack for brevity to shorten phrasing and simplify language. These individuals will strengthen the final product by trimming out the excess to highlight the essentials.

Once received, pool all feedback. Carefully consider which suggestions to incorporate in the rewrites, and which to exclude. Once all authors have authorized the changes to the manuscript, it is appropriate to submit.

Understand that manuscript submission is just the first step towards publication. There is no guarantee that submission will lead to publication, and even if it does, recognize that there is a long road ahead.

14.9 The Road to Publication

The road to publication is only just beginning with manuscript submission. Submission opens up your writing to extensive peer review. Peer review may be intimidating, but the intent is constructive. The majority of peer reviewers are volunteers. They expend a fair amount of energy on their own time because they want to.

Think of manuscript reviewers as having a stake in what the journal produces and in how you represent yourself. These are experts who care about the content area and care about you. They evaluate submissions to determine whether they are publishable and if so, whether improvements are necessary to make them print-ready.

To assess your work, reviewers will consider if the material is: (1)

- Original
- Relevant
- Timely

- Scientific
- Clear
- Accurate

- Valid
- Appropriate.

Ultimately, peer reviewers will make a recommendation to the editor based upon their evaluation of the manuscript as a whole. Recommendations may be to: (1)

- Accept the article, as is, for publication
- Accept the article for publication, contingent on minor revisions
- Request minor revisions, then re-examine
- Request major revisions, then re-examine
- Reject the manuscript.

Be prepared for more than one round of revision. Manuscript revisions are processes that strengthen manuscript quality, content, and presentation. Working through manuscript revisions is one of the best ways to grow as a researcher and scientific author.

In the event that manuscripts are rejected, consider the reasons for rejection with objectivity rather than your gut response.

It may be that the manuscript: (1)

* Was poorly written
* Was built around a study design with fatal flaws
* Did not meet journal guidelines with regards to format, content, or category of submission
* Did not provide guarantee of IACUC or IRB approval
* Did not contribute new or original findings to the veterinary medical literature.

Rejections are a learning opportunity. They may be the end of the road for that one manuscript, but do not let them end your efforts to produce scientific writing.

The evolution of veterinary medicine depends upon your tenacity in the world of research to pioneer, design, and implement studies that think outside the box and add value or knowledge to the field.

END-OF-CHAPTER SUMMARY

Original research articles typically follow the structure that is outlined below:

* Introduction
* Methods
* Results
* Discussion.

The acronym, IMRaD, helps you to remember this structure. Although each journal's guidelines may require you to adjust this structure to match its expectations, IMRaD provides an organizational template to assist you with writing.

Every aspect of the article, from title to list of references, must be well executed.

Titles should be concise and accurately reflect both the content of the manuscript and its conclusions. Titles also often make reference to study design.

Key words or phrases augment the title and provide searchable clauses by which colleagues can find your article when inputting their query into a database.

The introduction is a brief description that sets the stage for the rest of the report. Think of the introduction as the top of an inverted pyramid: it begins broadly, then funnels in to narrow the topic towards the research question.

Once the research question has been identified in writing, the introduction outlines the hypothesis of the author(s) as well as the objectives of the study.

If the purpose of the introduction is to establish the research question, then the purpose of the materials and methods section is to explain how the author(s) set about to answer the question.

The materials and methods section must provide sufficient detail so that, if desired, readers could recreate the experiment. Flowcharts and other organizational diagrams may be needed to clarify complex study designs.

The materials and methods section must also clearly describe how the research data was analyzed.

The results section outlines the answer(s) that arose from conducting the experiment. Data may be consolidated in figures or tables.

The discussion section provides an interpretation of the data.

The abstract is typically written last, to reflect the tone, quality, content, and voice of the final draft of the manuscript. It must function as a stand-alone synopsis. The greatest challenge in writing the abstract is its limited word count. There is much to cover, but only a fraction can be included.

References

1. Christopher M, Young K. Writing for Publication in Veterinary Medicine: A Practical Guide for Researchers and Clinicians; 2015. Available from: http://www.wiley.com/legacy/wiley blackwell/gmspdfs/VETWritingforPub/pubData/source/VETWritingforPubPDF.pdf
2. Taylor RB. The Clinician's Guide to Medical Writing. New York: Springer; 2005. xiv, 266 pp.
3. Franklin SP, Burke EE, Holmes SP. The effect of platelet-rich plasma on osseous healing in dogs undergoing high tibial osteotomy. PLoS One. 2017;12(5):e0177597.
4. Nishimura LT, Villela IOJ, Carvalho LL, Borges LPB, Silva MAM, Mattos-Junior E. The effect of acepromazine alone or in combination with methadone, morphine, or tramadol on sedation and selected cardiopulmonary variables in sheep. Vet Med Int. 2017;2017:7507616.
5. Moore KL, Mullan BP, Kim JC, Payne HG, Dunshea FR. Effect of feed restriction and initial body weight on growth performance, body composition, and hormones in male pigs immunized against gonadotropin-releasing factor. J Anim Sci. 2016;94(9):3966–3977.
6. Calzetta L, Soggiu A, Roncada P, Bonizzi L, Pistocchini E, Urbani A, et al. Propofol protects against opioid-induced hyperresponsiveness of airway smooth muscle in a horse model of target-controlled infusion anaesthesia. Eur J Pharmacol. 2015;765:463–471.
7. Bol S, Bunnik EM. Lysine supplementation is not effective for the prevention or treatment of feline herpesvirus 1 infection in cats: a systematic review. BMC Vet Res. 2015;11:284.
8. Li Y, Ding H, Wang X, Liu L, Huang D, Zhang R, et al. High levels of acetoacetate and glucose increase expression of cytokines in bovine hepatocytes, through activation of the NF-κB signalling pathway. J Dairy Res. 2016;83(1):51–57.
9. Hamood WJ, Chur-Hansen A, McArthur ML. A qualitative study to explore communication skills in veterinary medical education. Int J Med Educ. 2014;5:193–198.

10. Englar RE, Williams M, Weingand K. Applicability of the Calgary-Cambridge Guide to dog and cat owners for teaching veterinary clinical communications. J Vet Med Educ. 2016;43(2):143–169.

11. Meyer B, Zentek J, Harlander-Matauschek A. Differences in intestinal microbial metabolites in laying hens with high and low levels of repetitive feather-pecking behavior. Physiol Behav. 2013;110–111:96–101.

12. Payne JR, Borgeat K, Brodbelt DC, Connolly DJ, Luis Fuentes V. Risk factors associated with sudden death vs. congestive heart failure or arterial thromboembolism in cats with hypertrophic cardiomyopathy. J Vet Cardiol. 2015;17 Suppl 1:S318–28.

13. Payne JR, Borgeat K, Connolly DJ, Boswood A, Dennis S, Wagner T, et al. Prognostic indicators in cats with hypertrophic cardiomyopathy. J Vet Inter Med. 2013;27(6):1427–1436.

14. Fuentes VL. Arterial thromboembolism: risks, realities and a rational first-line approach. J Feline Med Surg. 2012;14(7):459–470.

15. Information on Protection of Human Subjects in Research Funded or Regulated by U.S. Government: U.S. Department of Health and Human Services. Available from: https://www.hhs.gov/1946inoculationstudy/protection.html

16. Research Involving Human Participants, Human Material or Personal Data: UK Research Integrity Office. Available from: http://ukrio.org/publications/code-of-practice-for-research/3-0-standards-for-organisations-and-researchers/3-7-research-involving-human-participants-human-material-or-personal-data/

17. Martin WE, Bridgmon KD. Quantitative and Statistical Research Methods: from Hypothesis to Results. 1st ed. San Francisco: Jossey-Bass; 2012. xviii, 476 pp.

18. Creswell JW. Qualitative Inquiry & Research Design: Choosing Among Five Approaches. 2nd ed. Thousand Oaks, CA: Sage Publications; 2007. xvii, 395 pp.

19. Merriam SB, Tisdell EJ. Qualitative Research: A Guide to Design and Implementation. 4th edition. San Francisco, CA: Jossey-Bass; 2016. xix, 346 pp.

Appendix 1

Supplemental Exercises to Master Veterinary Medical Jargon

For practice purposes following your review of Chapter 2, answer key from page 212.

Exercise 1: Recalling Roots

Write the meaning of the roots provided below:

1. Nephr(o)- . . . .
2. Cyst- . . . .
3. Hepat(o)- . . . .
4. Stomat(o)- . . . .
5. Bucc- . . . .
6. Onych(o)- . . . .
7. Blephar(o)- . . . .
8. Odont(o)- . . . .
9. Lingu(a)- . . . .
10. Thorac(o)- . . . .

Exercise 2: Recalling Roots

Provide the root(s) for the body parts that are listed below:

1. Hair . . . .
2. Gland . . . .
3. Blood . . . .
4. Lungs . . . .
5. Ear . . . .
6. Bone . . . .
7. Gall bladder . . . .
8. Head . . . .
9. Heart . . . .
10. Gums . . . .

Exercise 3: Recalling Roots

Write the meaning of the roots provided below:

1. Encephal(o)- . . . .
2. Mast- . . . .
3. Orchid(o)- . . . .
4. Labi(o)- . . . .
5. Vesic- . . . .
6. Dors- . . . .
7. Oculo- . . . .
8. Umbilic- . . . .
9. Cost(o)- . . . .
10. Om(o)- . . . .

Exercise 4: Recalling Roots

Provide the root(s) for the body parts that are listed below:

1. Abdomen . . . .
2. Hip . . . .
3. Intestine . . . .
4. Muscle . . . .
5. Nose . . . .
6. Rib . . . .
7. Navel . . . .
8. Skin . . . .
9. Neck . . . .
10. Bone marrow . . . .

Exercise 5: Recalling Prefixes

Write the meaning of the prefixes provided below:

1. Aniso- . . . .
2. Axill- . . . .
3. Brachy- . . . .
4. Brady- . . . .
5. Hemi- . . . .
6. Acro- . . . .
7. Allo- . . . .
8. Chemo- . . . .
9. Ventr(o)- . . . .
10. Xen(o)- . . . .
11. Amphi- . . . .

12. An- . . . .

13. Cata- . . . .

14. Tetra- . . . .

15. Contra- . . . .

Exercise 6: Recalling Prefixes

Write the prefix(es) that match(es) the meaning given below:

1. Blood vessel . . . .

2. Joints. . . . .

3. Below . . . .

4. Between . . . .

5. Behind . . . .

6. Fast. . . . .

7. Up, above. . . . .

8. Tears . . . .

9. Crooked . . . .

10. Bad, ill . . . .

11. Large. . . . .

12. In front of . . . .

13. One . . . .

14. Self . . . .

15. Spine . . . .

Exercise 7: Recalling Suffixes

Write the meaning of the suffixes provided below:

1. -asthenia . . . .
2. -dactyl . . . .
3. -dynia . . . .
4. -gnosis . . . .
5. -iasis . . . .
6. -malacia . . . .
7. -penia . . . .
8. -pexy . . . .
9. -oma . . . .
10. -pathy . . . .

Exercise 8: Recalling Suffixes

Write the suffix that matches the word description below:

1. Enzyme . . . .
2. Hardening . . . .
3. To secrete . . . .
4. Stopping . . . .
5. Resembling . . . .
6. Cutting . . . .
7. Production . . . .
8. Spitting . . . .
9. Contraction . . . .
10. Thirst . . . .

Exercise 9: Recalling Suffixes

Write the meaning of the suffixes provided below:

1. -cidal . . . .

2. -pepsia . . . .

3. -lysis . . . .

4. -phil(ia) . . . .

5. -phagia . . . .

6. -lepsy . . . .

7. -stomy . . . .

8. -tripsy . . . .

9. -ptosis . . . .

10. -spadias . . . .

Exercise 10: Recalling Suffixes

Write the suffix that matches the word description below:

1. Pouching, hernia. . . . .

2. Suturing . . . .

3. Turning . . . .

4. Development . . . .

5. Formation . . . .

6. Pricking . . . .

7. Image, record . . . .

8. Condition of . . . .

9. Knowledge . . . .

10. Fixation. . . . .

Exercise 11: Putting It All Together

Use your knowledge of prefixes, roots, and suffixes to translate the following medical jargon into everyday language:

1. Cholecystectomy . . . .
2. Colostomy . . . .
3. Onychectomy . . . .
4. Thoracotomy . . . .
5. Bronchoscopy . . . .
6. Arthropathy . . . .
7. Anesthesia . . . .
8. Gastropexy . . . .
9. Trichogram . . . .
10. Laparoscopy . . . .

Exercise 12: Putting It All Together

Use your knowledge of prefixes, roots, and suffixes to translate the following everyday language into medical jargon:

1. The study of the heart . . . .
2. The study of skin . . . .
3. Viewing the nose with an instrument . . . .
4. Stopping blood . . . .
5. Viewing the urinary bladder with an instrument . . . .
6. Half paralysis . . . .
7. Suturing of the eyelid . . . .
8. Softening of the brain tissue . . . .
9. Inflammation of the bone . . . .
10. Without development . . . .

Exercise 13: Putting It All Together

Use your knowledge of prefixes, roots, and suffixes to translate the following medical jargon into everyday language:

1. Renomegaly . . . .
2. Odontalgia . . . .
3. Megacolon . . . .
4. Cholecystitis . . . .
5. Microhepatica. . . . .
6. Tachypnea . . . .
7. Bradycardia . . . .
8. Hemoptysis. . . . .
9. Brachycephalic. . . . .
10. Orchitis. . . . .

Exercise 14: Putting It All Together

Use your knowledge of prefixes, roots, and suffixes to translate the following everyday language into medical jargon:

1. The study of the kidney. . . . .
2. Difficulty with urination . . . .
3. Inflammation of the nose . . . .
4. Difficulty with breathing . . . .
5. Inflammation of the urinary bladder . . . .
6. Painful muscles. . . . .
7. Transfusion with blood from another species. . . . .
8. Muscle weakness . . . .
9. Breakdown of bone. . . . .
10. Disease of nerves . . . .

Exercise 15: Putting It All Together: Procedures

Use your knowledge of prefixes, roots, and suffixes to translate the following medical jargon into everyday language:

1. Ophthalmoscopy . . . .

2. Splenectomy . . . .

3. Arthroscopy . . . .

4. Laparoscopy . . . .

5. Herniorrhaphy . . . .

6. Otoscopy . . . .

7. Thoracocentesis . . . .

8. Cystotomy . . . .

9. Gastrotomy . . . .

10. Celiotomy . . . .

Exercise 16: Putting It All Together: Procedures II

Use your knowledge of prefixes, roots, and suffixes to translate the following medical jargon into everyday language:

1. Ovariohysterectomy . . . .

2. Ostectomy . . . .

3. Tracheostomy . . . .

4. Urethrostomy . . . .

5. Colectomy . . . .

6. Pericardiocentesis . . . .

7. Enterotomy . . . .

8. Colonoscopy . . . .

9. Abdominocentesis . . . .

10. Cholecystectomy . . . .

Exercise 17: Putting It All Together: Specialty Areas of Medical Study

Use your knowledge of prefixes, roots, and suffixes to translate the following medical jargon into everyday language:

1. Cardiology . . . .

2. Oncology . . . .

3. Hematology . . . .

4. Ophthalmology. . . . .

5. Pathology . . . .

6. Neurology. . . . .

7. Microbiology . . . .

8. Endocrinology. . . . .

9. Dermatology. . . . .

10. Arthrology. . . . .

Exercise 18: Putting It All Together: Terms That Describe Pathology

Use your knowledge of prefixes, roots, and suffixes to translate the following medical jargon into everyday language:

1. Dyspepsia. . . . .

2. Dysuria. . . . .

3. Dyspnea . . . .

4. Dysfunction . . . .

5. Dysphagia. . . . .

6. Dysplasia . . . .

7. Dyschezia. . . . .

8. Dyskinesia . . . .

9. Dystrophy. . . . .

10. Dysphoria. . . . .

Exercise 19: Putting It All Together: Terms That Describe Pathology II

Use your knowledge of prefixes, roots, and suffixes to translate the following medical jargon into everyday language:

1. Hematoma . . . .

2. Sarcoma . . . .

3. Neuroma . . . .

4. Lymphoma . . . .

5. Adenoma . . . .

6. Lipoma . . . .

7. Chondroma. . . . .

8. Myeloma . . . .

9. Meningioma. . . . .

10. Melanoma . . . .

Exercise 20: Putting It All Together: Terms That Describe Pathology III

Use your knowledge of prefixes, roots, and suffixes to translate the following medical jargon into everyday language:

1. Osteitis . . . .

2. Blepharitis. . . . .

3. Colitis. . . . .

4. Orchitis. . . . .

5. Nephritis. . . . .

6. Arthritis. . . . .

7. Bronchitis . . . .

8. Mastitis. . . . .

9. Dacryocystitis. . . . .

10. Adenitis . . . .

Exercise 21: Putting It All Together: Terms That Describe Pathology IV

Use your knowledge of prefixes, roots, and suffixes to translate the following medical jargon into everyday language:

1. Cardiomegaly . . . .

2. Microcardia . . . .

3. Dactylomegaly . . . .

4. Gastromegaly . . . .

5. Adrenomegaly . . . .

6. Megacolon . . . .

7. Microphthalmia . . . .

8. Megaesophagus . . . .

9. Renomegaly . . . .

10. Hepatomegaly . . . .

Exercise 22: Completing Medical Sentences

Use your knowledge of prefixes, roots, and suffixes to replace the italicized phrase with the medical term that most appropriately completes the meaning of the sentence:

1. The dog presented with bilaterally symmetrical temporal muscle *wasting*. . . . .
. . . .

2. Based upon physical exam findings, the cat has *enlarged kidneys*. . . . .
. . . .

3. The radiograph of the dog's distal femur shows *destruction of the bone* . . . .
. . . .

4. The racehorse was diagnosed with *inflammation of a tendon and its sheath* . . . . . .
. . . .

5. There is a mass that is *behind the eyeball* . . . .
. . . .

6. The cat's neck is *tucked to the chest* . . . .
. . . .

7. To prevent gastric dilatation-volvulus (GDV), the stomach undergoes *tacking to the body wall* . . . .

8. To look for evidence of an ectopic ureter, the dog needs to undergo *scoping of the urinary bladder* . . . .

9. On physical exam, a large *armpit* mass was identified. . . . .

10. Following *surgical removal of the front claws,* the cat developed an infection. . . . .

Exercise 23: Completing Medical Sentences

Use your knowledge of prefixes, roots, and suffixes to translate the medical jargon that has been italicized into everyday language that most appropriately completes the meaning of the sentence:

1. The intact female dog presented with *pyometra* . . . .

2. The dachshund's severe dental disease has resulted in *halitosis* . . . .

3. After eating a block of cheddar cheese and Swedish meatballs, the dog presented for *dyspepsia* . . . .

4. The corneal ulcer has caused the patient to exhibit *photophobia* . . . .

5. On physical examination, the cat is *polydactyl*: she has seven toes on each front foot and five on each back. . . . .

6. An abdominal *radiograph* demonstrated the cause of the urinary obstruction . . . .

7. *Urolithiasis* is a concern particularly in a male cat . . . .

8. The patient's comprehensive blood count demonstrates *neutrophilia* . . . .

9. The severity of the cat's *stomatitis* has caused him to be anorexic. . . . .

10. Because the dog is *brachycephalic,* additional precautions will need to be taken when she is anesthetized . . . .

Exercise 24: Directional Terms

Match each directional term that is listed below in the left-hand column with the appropriate definition in the right-hand column:

A.	Abaxial	1. Towards the back.
B.	Adaxial	2. Towards the breastbone.
C.	Cranial	3. Near the surface of the patient's skin.
D.	Caudal	4. Towards the belly.
E.	Deep	5. Towards the braincase.
F.	Distal	6. Away from a limb's longitudinal central axis.
G.	Dorsal	7. The surface of a paw that touches the ground.
H.	Lateral	8. Towards a limb's longitudinal central axis.
I.	Medial	9. Towards the tail.
J.	Plantar	10. Away from midline.
K.	Proximal	11. Towards the nose or beak.
L.	Rostral	12. Towards midline.
M.	Sternal	13. Away from the trunk.
N.	Superficial	14. Away from/underneath the skin, nearer to the patient's core.
O.	Ventral	15. Towards the trunk.

Exercise 25: Anatomical Planes

Match each anatomical plane that is listed below in the left-hand column with the appropriate definition in the right-hand column:

A.	Dorsal	1. This plane divides the body into *equal* right and left parts.
B.	Median	2. This plane is parallel to the back.
C.	Sagittal	3. This plane is perpendicular to the long axis of the patient and divides the body into cranial and caudal halves.
D.	Transverse	4. This plane divides the body into right and left parts.

Exercise 26: Anatomical Adjectives

Match each anatomical adjective that is listed below in the left-hand column with the body part that it describes in the right-hand column:

A.	Antebrachial	1. Heel
B.	Aural	2. Neck
C.	Axillary	3. Rib
D.	Brachial	4. Finger or toe
E.	Buccal	5. Tongue
F.	Calcaneal	6. Eye
G.	Carpal	7. Groin
H.	Cephalic	8. Back of the elbow
I.	Cervical	9. Armpit
J.	Crural	10. Lower back
K.	Costal	11. Between the pubic symphysis and the coccyx
L.	Coccygeal	12. Head
M.	Coxal	13. Ankle
N.	Digital	14. Back of knee
O.	Femoral	15. Upper arm
P.	Gluteal	16. Tailbone
Q.	Inguinal	17. Foot
R.	Labial	18. Ear
S.	Lingual	19. Hip
T.	Lumbar	20. Wrist
U.	Occipital	21. Hoof, nail, or claw
V.	Ocular	22. Forearm
W.	Olecranal	23. Thigh
X.	Patellar	24. Knee cap
Y.	Pedal	25. Chest
Z.	Perineal	26. Skull base
AA.	Popliteal	27. Lip
BB.	Sacral	28. Lower leg
CC.	Tarsal	29. Buttocks
DD.	Thoracic	30. Base of the spine
EE.	Ungual	31. Cheek

Exercise 27: Reviewing Veterinary Medical Abbreviations: Pharmacy

Match each veterinary medical abbreviation that is listed below in the left-hand column with the definition that it describes in the right-hand column:

A.	BID	1.	As needed
B.	EOW	2.	Every other day
C.	QOD	3.	Twice a day
D.	TID	4.	Every other week
E.	Bol	5.	Four times a day
F.	QD	6.	Every day
G.	PRN	7.	Bolus
H.	QID	8.	Three times a day

Exercise 28: Reviewing Veterinary Medical Abbreviations: Body Parts

Provide the veterinary medical abbreviation that is the best substitute for the italicized word(s) in the sentences below:

1. The intact female dog presented with blepharospasm of *the right eye.* . . . .
    . . . .

2. The Dachshund's severe otitis externa is unilateral: it involves only *the left ear.* . . . .
    . . . .

3. The kitten has developed green purulent discharge in *both eyes.* . . . .
    . . . .

4. *Both ears* are infested with ear mites. . . . .
    . . . .

5. The Scottish Fold cat's *right ear* has developed an aural hematoma. . . . .
    . . . .

6. The cat's *left eye* is afflicted with an iris melanoma. . . . .
    . . . .

Exercise 29: Identifying Body Parts on a Feline Diagram

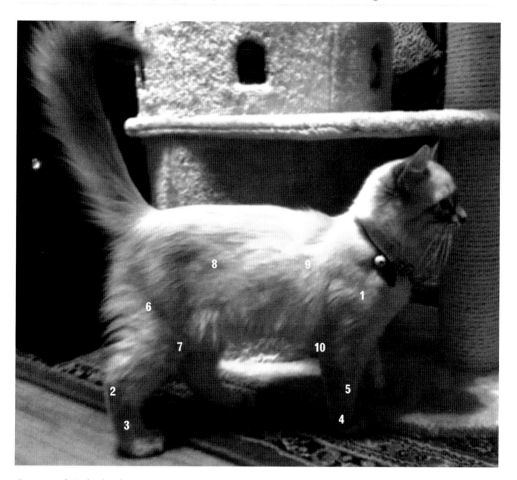

Courtesy of Kimberly Alvarez

Identify the body name or region that matches each number listed on the diagram above:

1. . . . .   6. . . . .

2. . . . .   7. . . . .

3. . . . .   8. . . . .

4. . . . .   9. . . . .

5. . . . .   10. . . . .

Exercise 30: Identifying Body Parts on an Equine Diagram

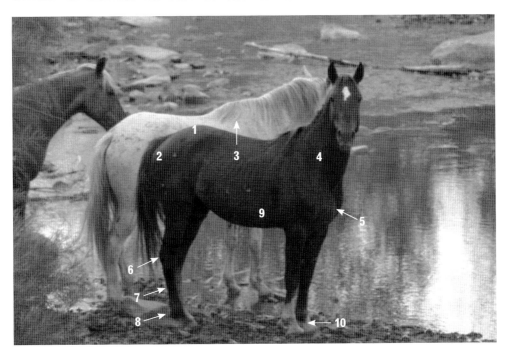

Courtesy of Laura Polerecky

Identify the body name or region that matches each number listed on the diagram above:

1. . . . .   6. . . . .

2. . . . .   7. . . . .

3. . . . .   8. . . . .

4. . . . .   9. . . . .

5. . . . .   10. . . . .

Exercise 31: Identifying Body Parts on a Bovine Diagram

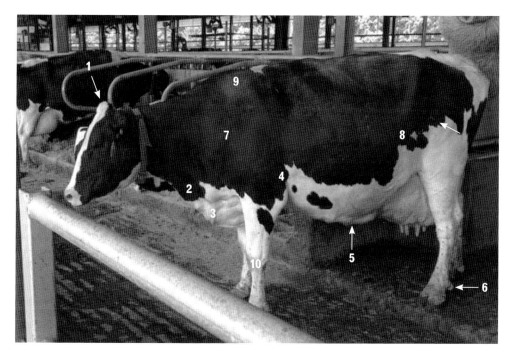

Courtesy of Tradel Harris, DVM

Identify the body name or region that matches each number listed on the diagram above:

1. . . . .   6. . . . .

2. . . . .   7. . . . .

3. . . . .   8. . . . .

4. . . . .   9. . . . .

5. . . . .   10. . . . .

Answer Key to Exercises

Exercise 1: Recalling Roots

1. Kidney
2. Bladder
3. Liver
4. Mouth
5. Cheek
6. Nail
7. Eyelid
8. Tooth
9. Tongue
10. Chest or rib cage

Exercise 2: Recalling Roots

1. Trich(o)-, capill-
2. Aden(o)-
3. Hem-, hemat-, sangui-, sanguine-
4. Pneumon-, pulmo-, pulmon(i)-
5. Ot(o)-, aur(i)-
6. Oste-, ossi-
7. Cholecyst(o)-, fell-
8. Cephal(o)-, capit(o)-
9. Cardi(o)-, cordi-
10. Gingiv-

Exercise 3: Recalling Roots

1. Brain
2. Breast
3. Testis
4. Lip
5. Urinary bladder
6. Back
7. Eye
8. Navel
9. Rib
10. Shoulder

Exercise 4: Recalling Roots

1. Lapar-, abdomin-
2. Cox-
3. Enter(o)-
4. My(o)-
5. Rhin(o)-, nas-
6. Pleur(o)-, cost(o)-
7. Omphal(o)-, umbilic-
8. Dermat(o)-, derm-, cut-, cuticul-
9. Trachel(o)-, cervic-
10. Myel-, medull-

Exercise 5: Recalling Prefixes

1. Not the same; unequal
2. Related to the armpit
3. Short
4. Slow
5. Half
6. Extreme
7. Other; Different
8. Drug
9. Belly
10. Foreign
11. Both sides
12. Without
13. Down, under
14. Four
15. Against

Exercise 6: Recalling Prefixes

1. Angi-
2. Arthr-
3. Hypo-
4. Inter-
5. Retro-
6. Tachy-
7. Epi-
8. Dacryo-
9. Ankyl(o)-
10. Dys-
11. Macro-
12. Pre-
13. Uni-
14. Auto-
15. Acantho-

Exercise 7: Recalling Suffixes

1. Weakness
2. Pertaining to toes
3. Pain
4. Knowledge
5. Condition of
6. Softening
7. Deficiency
8. Fixation
9. Tumor
10. Condition or disease

Exercise 8: Recalling Suffixes

1. -ase
2. -sclerosis
3. -crine
4. -stasis
5. -oid
6. -tomy
7. -poiesis
8. -ptysis
9. -stalsis
10. -dipsia

Exercise 9: Recalling Suffixes

1. Killing
2. Related to digestion
3. Separation
4. Attraction for
5. Related to ingestion
6. Attack
7. To create an opening
8. Crushing
9. Droopy
10. Fissure

Exercise 10: Recalling Suffixes

1. -cele
2. -rrhaphy
3. -version
4. -trophy
5. -plasia

6. -centesis
7. -gram
8. -iasis
9. -gnosis
10. -pexy

Exercise 11: Putting It All Together

1. Cutting out the gall bladder
2. Creating an opening in the colon
3. Cutting out the nail or claw
4. Cutting into the rib cage or chest
5. Viewing of the lungs with an instrument
6. Disease of the joints
7. Without sensation
8. Fixation of the stomach
9. Image of hair
10. Viewing the abdomen with an instrument

Exercise 12: Putting It All Together

1. Cardiology
2. Dermatology
3. Rhinoscopy
4. Hemostasis
5. Cystoscopy

6. Hemiplegia
7. Tarsorrhaphy
8. Encephalomalacia
9. Osteitis
10. Atrophy

Exercise 13: Putting It All Together

1. Enlarged kidneys
2. Tooth pain
3. Enlarged colon
4. Inflammation of the gall bladder
5. Small liver

6. Increased respiration
7. Decreased heart rate
8. Coughing up blood
9. Short-faced
10. Inflammation of the testicles

Exercise 14: Putting It All Together

1. Nephrology
2. Dysuria
3. Rhinitis
4. Dyspnea
5. Cystitis
6. Myalgia
7. Xenotransfusion
8. Myasthenia
9. Osteolysis
10. Neuropathy

Exercise 15: Putting It All Together

1. Viewing or scoping of the eye
2. Surgical removal of the spleen
3. Viewing or scoping of the joints
4. Viewing or scoping of the abdomen
5. Suturing of a hernia
6. Viewing or scoping of the ear
7. Sticking a needle into the thoracic cavity
8. Cutting into the urinary bladder
9. Cutting into the stomach
10. Cutting into the abdominal cavity

Exercise 16: Putting It All Together

1. Surgical removal of the ovaries and uterus
2. Surgical removal of bone
3. Cutting into the trachea
4. Cutting into the urethra
5. Surgical removal of the colon or a portion of the colon
6. Sticking a needle into the pericardial sac
7. Cutting into the intestine
8. Viewing or scoping of the colon
9. Sticking a needle into the abdominal cavity
10. Surgical removal of the gall bladder

Exercise 17: Putting It All Together: Specialty Areas of Medical Study

1. The study of the heart
2. The study of tumors
3. The study of blood
4. The study of eyes
5. The study of disease
6. The study of the nervous system
7. The study of microorganisms
8. The study of hormones
9. The study of skin
10. The study of joints

Exercise 18: Putting It All Together: Terms That Describe Pathology

1. "Bad stomach" – i.e. upset stomach
2. Difficult urination
3. Difficulty breathing
4. Abnormal function
5. Difficulty swallowing
6. Abnormal growth
7. Difficult defecation
8. Abnormal voluntary movement
9. Abnormal degeneration of tissue
10. Abnormal state of being; extreme state of unease

Exercise 19: Putting It All Together: Terms That Describe Pathology II

1. Tumor of clotted blood
2. Tumor of connective tissue, such as muscle
3. Thickening of nerve tissue
4. Cancer of the immune system
5. Tumor of glandular tissue
6. Tumor of fat
7. Tumor of cartilage
8. Cancer of plasma cells
9. Tumor of the meninges
10. One type of skin cancer involving the pigment-producing cells

Exercise 20: Putting It All Together: Terms That Describe Pathology III

1. Inflammation of the bone
2. Inflammation of the eyelids
3. Inflammation of the colon
4. Inflammation of the testicle
5. Inflammation of the kidney
6. Inflammation of the joints
7. Inflammation of the bronchial tubes
8. Inflammation of breast tissue
9. Inflammation of the lacrimal sac
10. Inflammation of glandular tissue

Exercise 21: Putting It All Together: Terms That Describe Pathology IV

1. Enlarged heart
2. Abnormally small heart
3. Abnormally enlarged digit
4. Enlarged stomach
5. Enlarged adrenal gland
6. Enlarged colon
7. Abnormally small eye
8. Enlarged esophagus
9. Enlarged kidney
10. Enlarged liver

Exercise 22: Completing Medical Sentences

1. Atrophy
2. Renomegaly
3. Osteolysis
4. Tenosynovitis
5. Retro-orbital
6. Ventroflexed
7. Gastropexy
8. Cystoscopy
9. Axillary
10. Onychectomy

Exercise 23: Completing Medical Sentences

1. Pus in the uterus/uterine infection
2. Bad breath
3. Upset stomach
4. Light-fearing/light sensitivity
5. Extra-toed
6. X-ray image
7. Bladder stones
8. Increased white blood cells/increased neutrophils
9. Mouth infection
10. Short-faced

Exercise 24: Directional Terms

1. G
2. M
3. N
4. O
5. C
6. A
7. J
8. B
9. D
10. H
11. L
12. I
13. F
14. E
15. K

Exercise 25: Anatomical Planes

1. B
2. A
3. D
4. C

Exercise 26: Anatomical Adjectives

1. F	8. W	15. D	22. A	29. P
2. I	9. C	16. L	23. O	30. BB
3. K	10. T	17. Y	24. X	31. E
4. N	11. Z	18. B	25. DD	
5. S	12. H	19. M	26. U	
6. V	13. CC	20. G	27. R	
7. Q	14. AA	21. EE	28. J	

Exercise 27: Reviewing Veterinary Medical Abbreviations: Pharmacy

1. G	3. A	5. H	7. E
2. C	4. B	6. F	8. D

Exercise 28: Reviewing Veterinary Medical Abbreviations: Body Parts

1. OD	4. AU
2. AS	5. AD
3. OU	6. OS

Exercise 29: Identifying Body Parts on a Feline Diagram

1. Brachium	6. Upper thigh
2. Tarsus or hock	7. Stifle or knee
3. Metatarsus	8. Abdomen
4. Forepaw	9. Thorax
5. Antebrachium	10. Elbow

Exercise 30: Identifying Body Parts on an Equine Diagram

1. Croup	6. Hock
2. Buttock	7. Cannon
3. Withers	8. Fetlock
4. Neck	9. Barrel
5. Chest	10. Pastern

Exercise 31: Identifying Body Parts on a Bovine Diagram

1. Poll
2. Dewlap
3. Brisket
4. Elbow
5. Milk veins

6. Dewclaw
7. Shoulder
8. Flank
9. Withers
10. Knee

Appendix 2

Supplemental Exercises to Master the Medical Record

For practice purposes following your review of Chapters 4–7, answer key from page 243

Exercise 1: History-Taking

History-taking requires you, the clinician, to obtain important details about patient health and lifestyle in order for you to conduct a thorough veterinary consultation. In order to take a comprehensive patient history, you need to ask a number of questions. Using the funnel approach and a mix of closed-ended and open-ended questions can be helpful.

The following statements and questions are items that you might choose to ask the client during history-taking.

Identify whether each statement or question is closed-ended (C) or open-ended (O) in the blank provided:

...... 1. Did Katniss eat breakfast this morning?

...... 2. Tell me everything that you feed Katniss.

...... 3. Describe Katniss' daily routine.

...... 4. When was the last time that Katniss ate?

...... 5. Did Katniss vomit after she ate last night?

...... 6. Did you see Bella collapse?

...... 7. Share with me what you saw Bella do when she had her last fainting episode.

...... 8. Describe what you notice once Bella gets back up after her episode.

...... 9. Does Bella seem blind after each episode?

...... 10. Did Bella lose control of her bladder when she fainted?

Exercise 2: Transforming Closed-Ended Questions into Open-Ended Questions or Statements

Although closed-ended questions are valuable in that they allow you, the clinician, to clarify key facts or details about patient health and lifestyle, it is often helpful for you to start with an open-ended question. This invites the client to share his/her perspective with you and the rest of the veterinary team. The client is likely to provide you with more information than you may have obtained had you led with a closed-ended question.

The following questions are closed-ended.

Transform each into an open-ended question or statement:

. . . . . . 1. Is Edward energetic?

. . . . . . 2. What do you feed Edward?

. . . . . . 3. Do you apply flea/tick preventative to Edward?

. . . . . . 4. Is Edward up-to-date on vaccinations?

. . . . . . 5. Do you bathe Edward?

. . . . . . 6. Where did you get Peeta?

. . . . . . 7. Have you noticed blood in Peeta's urine?

. . . . . . 8. Has Peeta been straining to urinate?

. . . . . . 9. Is Peeta eating?

. . . . . . 10. Is Peeta exposed to other cats?

Exercise 3: A Detailed Approach to History-Taking

History-taking is an opportunity for the client to share information with you, the clinician, and the rest of the veterinary team. Not all clients choose to share the same amount of information. Many require follow-up questions to clarify and/or obtain additional details.

The following statements are answers that clients provided when you took a patient history.

For each statement, identify at least two details that are missing that require follow-up questions:

1. I feed Carmello twice a day . . . .
. . . .

2. I give Fiji flea/tick preventative . . . .
. . . .

3. Tulip is up-to-date on vaccinations . . . .
    . . . .

4. When we adopted Christopher, we were told that he was healthy. . . . .
    . . . .

5. I scoop the litter box every other day . . . .
    . . . .

Exercise 4: Breaking Down the "S" in SOAP

The following phrases are typical of those obtained during history-taking. Each statement needs to be included in the "S" of the SOAP note. Write the letter of each phrase in the blank following the appropriate header where the statement would best belong in the "S."

Headers

1. Demographic data: . . . .

2. Presenting complaint: . . . .

3. Lifestyle and activity level: . . . .

4. Travel history: . . . .

5. Serologic status: . . . .

6. Diet history: . . . .

7. Vaccination history: . . . .

8. Past pertinent medical history: . . . .

Phrases

A. FVRCP vaccinations were discontinued four years ago
B. Female spayed
C. Feline leukemia (FeLV) negative
D. History of antibiotic-responsive diarrhea two years ago
E. Indoor/outdoor
F. Cheddar cheese treats
G. Feline immunodeficiency virus (FIV) negative
H. Receives monthly topical flea/tick preventative

I.   12-year-old
J.   Sleeps 18 hours/day
K.   Defecated today on the foyer carpet
L.   Receives glucosamine-chondroitin supplement daily
M.   Up-to-date on rabies vaccination
N.   Urinated next to litter box yesterday
O.   Ragdoll cat
P.   Canned tuna fish in oil once/week
Q.   Travelled by car from Boulder, CO to Phoenix, AZ last week
R.   Commercial feline adult dry kibble 1/4 c BID

Exercise 5: Breaking Down the "S" in SOAP

The following phrases are typical of those obtained during history-taking. Each statement needs to be included in the "S" of the SOAP note. Write the letter of each phrase in the blank following the appropriate header where the statement would best belong in the "S."

Headers

1.   Demographic data: . . . .

2.   Presenting complaint: . . . .

3.   Lifestyle and activity level: . . . .

4.   Travel history: . . . .

5.   Serologic status: . . . .

6.   Diet history: . . . .

7.   Vaccination history: . . . .

8.   Past pertinent medical history: . . . .

Phrases

A.   Right forelimb lameness progressing to non-weight-bearing status today
B.   Home-cooked, raw beef, rolled into meatballs equivalent to 1/4 pound BID
C.   Treated for chocolate toxicosis at 6 months of age
D.   Agility training classes 2x/week
E.   Boiled whole grain rice

F.   Went to agility competition in Connecticut last month
G.   Client is concerned about borreliosis
H.   *Ehrlichia* negative on ELISA snap test
I.   Overdue on DH2PP
J.   Border Collie
K.   Doggie day care every Monday
L.   Excessively licking right carpus
M.   4-year-old
N.   Receives monthly topical heartworm preventative
O.   Otitis externa AU, successfully managed two summers ago
P.   Frozen snowpeas
Q.   Intact male
R.   Up-to-date on rabies vaccination

Exercise 6: Breaking Down the "S" in SOAP

The following phrases are typical of those obtained during history-taking. Each statement needs to be included in the "S" of the SOAP note. Write the letter of each phrase in the blank following the appropriate header where the statement would best belong in the "S."

Headers

1.   Demographic data: . . . .

2.   Presenting complaint: . . . .

3.   Lifestyle and activity level: . . . .

4.   Travel history: . . . .

5.   Serologic status: . . . .

6.   Diet history: . . . .

7.   Vaccination history: . . . .

8.   Past pertinent medical history: . . . .

Phrases

A. Negative Coggins test six months ago
B. Restless
C. 1/2 scoop of pelleted feed every morning
D. Quarter Horse
E. Trail rides every weekend
F. Annually vaccinated against tetanus
G. 7-year-old
H. Relocated to Virginia six months ago
I. Eats peppermints as treats
J. Pawing at the ground
K. 1 flake of alfalfa BID
L. Pleasure riding horse
M. Bout of medically managed colic last summer
N. Gelding
O. 1/4 c molasses every other day
P. Flank-watching
Q. Purchased from upstate New York
R. Bay

Exercise 7: Breaking Down the "S" in SOAP

The following phrases are typical of those obtained during history-taking. Each statement needs to be included in the "S" of the SOAP note. Write the letter of each phrase in the blank following the appropriate header where the statement would best belong in the "S."

Headers

1. Demographic data: . . . .

2. Presenting complaint: . . . .

3. Lifestyle, environment, and activity level: . . . .

4. Travel history: . . . .

5. Serologic status: . . . .

6. Diet history: . . . .

7. Vaccination history: . . . .

8. Past pertinent medical history: . . . .

Phrases

A. High-protein calf starter mix
B. Herd is seronegative for bovine leukemia virus (BLV)
C. Segregated by age
D. Holstein
E. Weak
F. Individually housed in plastic hutch
G. Orally vaccinated against bovine rotavirus and coronavirus as a newborn
H. Did not receive colostrum until 8+ hours after birth
I. Bull calf
J. IBR-BVD-PI3-BRSV vaccine was given at 8 weeks old
K. Yellow stool progressing to watery diarrhea overnight
L. 12% of calves last season had scours
M. Depressed
N. Blackleg 7-way vaccination was given at 8 weeks old
O. 11-day-old
P. Milk replacer
Q. Decreased appetite
R. Upstate New York dairy

Exercise 8: "S" vs. "O"

Indicate whether the following phrases belong in the "S" or the "O" portion of the SOAP:

Phrases

. . . . . . 1. Axillary papulopustular rash

. . . . . . 2. 4-year-old female spayed British Shorthair cat

. . . . . . 3. Adopted from a cattery last summer

. . . . . . 4. Positive menace response OU

. . . . . . 5. Non-reducible umbilical hernia

. . . . . . 6. Travels with owner by car between Georgia and North Carolina 2x/year

. . . . . . 7. History of FeLV/FIV neg/neg as a kitten

. . . . . . 8. Polydactyly – all four paws

. . . . . . 9. Acutely pruritic

. . . . . . 10. Grooming excessively since Saturday

Exercise 9: "S" vs. "O"

Indicate whether the following phrases belong in the "S" or the "O" portion of the SOAP:

Phrases

...... 1. Intermittent scooting since Sunday

...... 2. Three-week history of dyschezia

...... 3. Palpably enlarged, non-painful prostate

...... 4. Licking perineum excessively in owner's presence

...... 5. Enlarged right anal sac

...... 6. 8-year-old male intact German Shepherd dog

...... 7. Hyperreactive

...... 8. Left-sided perianal fistula

...... 9. Grade 2/6 left systolic murmur

...... 10. Vocalizes upon defecation

Exercise 10: "S" vs. "O"

Indicate whether the following phrases belong in the "S" or the "O" portion of the SOAP:

Phrases

...... 1. Basking area ranges in temperature from 90°F–100°F

...... 2. Deformed spinal column

...... 3. 9-month-old iguana

...... 4. On examination, there is a swollen, "pouty" appearance to lower jaw

...... 5. Eats primarily iceberg lettuce, tomato, and canned cat food

...... 6. Decreased appetite and lethargy

...... 7. Dehydration estimated at 5%

...... 8. Enclosure humidity is maintained at 75%

...... 9. Enclosure lights are turned off at night

...... 10. Bilateral forelimb tetany

Exercise 11: "S" vs. "O"

Indicate whether the following phrases belong in the "S" or the "O" portion of the SOAP:

Phrases

...... 1. Decreased appetite for the past two days

...... 2. Reduced airflow – R nostril only

...... 3. Restless overnight

...... 4. Normal bronchovesicular lung sounds on thoracic auscultation

...... 5. Dull percussion over the right maxillary sinus

...... 6. Honey-colored right nasal discharge developed last week

...... 7. Abnormal digital pulses

...... 8. Respiratory stertor audible on examination

...... 9. 11-year-old Arabian mare

...... 10. Teeth were routinely floated last month

Exercise 12: "S" vs. "O"

Write the letter of the one statement in each cluster of five that belongs in the "S" of the SOAP note rather than the "O":

...... 1.

    a.   Two-view radiographs of the right forelimb
    b.   Swollen right lateral elbow
    c.   Limping for two weeks
    d.   Palpable crepitus over the left thorax
    e.   Rx: Metronidazole 250 mg: give 1 tablet PO BID

...... 2.

    a.   Euhydrated
    b.   Ingested 10 ounces of dark chocolate last night around 10:00 p.m.
    c.   Placed IV catheter in the left cephalic vein
    d.   Admitted to hospital for 24-hour observation
    e.   Placed on "seizure watch"

...... 3.

    a. Rx: Vitamin K1
    b. PT and aPTT significantly prolonged
    c. Ecchymoses present throughout the gingiva and both medial thighs
    d. Epistaxis
    e. History of rodenticide ingestion

...... 4.

    a. Overgrown nails
    b. History of adverse reactions to vaccinations; requires pre-medication with diphenhydramine
    c. Medial patellar luxation – left pelvic limb – Grade 2
    d. Fecal analysis: no ova seen
    e. HW/L/E/A: negative

...... 5.

    a. Surrendered to shelter for inappropriate elimination
    b. Two-view abdominal radiographs: no uroliths seen
    c. Urinary catheter placed
    d. Spontaneous urethral spasms noted on physical examination
    e. Palpably firm, painful urinary bladder

Exercise 13: Conversion Factors for Body Weight as Listed in the "O" Section of SOAP Notes – Part 1

Body weight is a numerical value that should be included in every medical record for every patient visit.

Body weight may be written in either kilograms (kg) or pounds (lb). It is critical that the veterinarian be able to convert between units as needed using the appropriate conversion factors.

The following patient weights have been provided for you, the clinician, in pounds. Convert each body weight from pounds to kilograms:

1. 12.3 lb. . . . .

2. 5 lb . . . .

3. 25 lb . . . .

4. 2 lb . . . .

5. 8 lb . . . .

6. 75 lb . . . .

7. 125 lb . . . .

8. 156 lb . . . .

9. 82 lb . . . .

10. 64 lb . . . .

Exercise 14: Conversion Factors for Body Weight as Listed in the "O" Section of SOAP Notes – Part 2

Body weight is a numerical value that should be included in every medical record for every patient visit.

Body weight may be written in either kilograms (kg) or pounds (lb). It is critical that the veterinarian be able to convert between units as needed using the appropriate conversion factors.

The following patient weights have been provided for you, the clinician, in kilograms.

Convert each body weight from kilograms to pounds:

1. 13 kg. . . . .

2. 19 kg. . . . .

3. 23 kg. . . . .

4. 52 kg. . . . .

5. 5 kg. . . . .

6. 29 kg. . . . .

7. 64 kg. . . . .

8. 11 kg . . . .

9. 2 kg. . . . .

10. 38 kg. . . . .

Exercise 15: Conversion Factors for Body Weight as Listed in the "O" Section of SOAP Notes – Part 3

Body weight is a numerical value that should be included in every medical record for every patient visit.

Body weight may be written in either kilograms (kg) or pounds (lb). It is critical that the veterinarian be able to convert between units as needed using the appropriate conversion factors.

Sometimes we get so used to inputting numbers into calculators that we forget to think through the conversion to see if the answer that the calculator came up with is in fact logical.

Consider the following conversions.

Without doing the calculation, identify if the answer should be *higher* or *lower* than the value you started with.

1. Converting 2 kg into lb . . . .

2. Converting 16 kg into lb . . . .

3. Converting 23 lb into kg . . . .

4. Converting 12 kg into lb . . . .

5. Converting 52 kg into lb . . . .

6. Converting 43 lb into kg . . . .

7. Converting 18 lb into kg . . . .

8. Converting 67 lb into kg . . . .

9. Converting 7 kg into lb . . . .

10. Converting 32 lb into kg . . . .

Exercise 16: Breaking Down the "A" in SOAP

The following problems are typical of those that may be included in the "A" section of the SOAP. Each problem may have one or more pathophysiological mechanisms.
 Match the pathophysiological mechanisms with the problem that best fits.
 Note that a letter may be associated with more than one problem

Problems

1. Emesis ....

2. Anemia ....

3. Urinary tract obstruction (UTO) ....

4. Azotemia ....

5. Leukocytosis ....

Pathophysiological Mechanisms

A. Activation of 5-HT3 receptors
B. Pre-renal
C. Enteric nervous system
D. Increased destruction of red blood cells
E. Internal mechanical blockage (i.e. urethrolith)
F. Renal
G. External mechanical blockage (i.e. prostatomegaly)
H. Inflammation
I. Post-renal
J. Decreased production of new red blood cells
K. Infection
L. Centrally mediated, via the chemoreceptor trigger zone (CTZ)
M. Loss of erythrocytes

Exercise 17: Breaking Down the "A" in SOAP

The following problems are typical of those that may be included in the "A" section of the SOAP. Each problem may have one or more pathophysiological mechanisms.

Match the pathophysiological mechanisms with the problem that best fits.

Note that a letter may be associated with more than one problem

Problems

1. Stranguria . . . .

2. Hypercalcemia . . . .

3. Urinary incontinence . . . .

4. Fever . . . .

Pathophysiological Mechanisms

A. Autoimmune
B. Endocrine (i.e. hypoadrenocorticism)
C. Renal failure
D. Urinary tract infection
E. Malignancy
F. Environmental (i.e. heatstroke)
G. Spinal cord disease
H. Sterile cystitis
I. Structural, as from a weak urinary sphincter
J. Polydipsia
K. Toxicosis, as from *Cestrum diurnum*
L. Mechanical obstruction (i.e. stricture)
M. Infectious

Exercise 18: Breaking Down the "A" in SOAP

The following problems are typical of those that may be included in the "A" section of the SOAP. Each problem may have one or more pathophysiological mechanisms.

Match the pathophysiological mechanisms with the problem that best fits.

Note that a letter may be associated with more than one problem

Problems

1. Polydipsia . . . .

2. Regurgitation . . . .

3. Pruritus . . . .

4. Heart murmur . . . .

Pathophysiological Mechanisms

A. Food allergy
B. Congenital, as from a persistent right fourth aortic arch
C. Contact dermatitis
D. Psychogenic
E. Acquired, as from megaesophagus
F. Endocrinopathy, such as diabetes mellitus
G. Structural issue, as from valvular insufficiency
H. Environmental allergy
I. Physiological, as from anemia
J. Metabolic, such as renal disease
K. Physiological, as from fever
L. Ectoparasite infestation
M. Medication-induced, as from diuretics

Exercise 19: Breaking Down the "P" in SOAP

The following phrases are typical of those that may be included in the "P" section of the SOAP. Each phrase best fits under "Diagnostic Plan" or "Therapeutic Plan."

    Write the letter of each phrase under the Section of the "P" in SOAP where it belongs.

Phrases

A. Check blood glucose.
B. Offer water ad libitum.
C. Recheck PCV every 2 hours.
D. Assess electrolytes every 8 hours.
E. Pull food by 10 p.m. in anticipation of surgery tomorrow morning.
F. Measure intraocular pressure OU.
G. Perform a fecal analysis.

H. Repeat 3-view thoracic radiographs tomorrow morning.
I. Administer injectable ampicillin SQ.
J. Schedule abdominal ultrasound for this afternoon.
K. Prescribe famotidine (10 mg): 1/4 tab PO BID, 30 minutes prior to mealtime.
L. Install pheromone diffuser in the litter box room at home to see if doing so reduces house-soiling.

Section of the "P" in SOAP

1. Diagnostic plan . . . .
2. Therapeutic plan . . . .

Exercise 20: Breaking Down the "P" in SOAP

The following phrases are typical of those that may be included in the "P" section of the SOAP. Each phrase best fits under "Diagnostic Plan" or "Therapeutic Plan."

   Write the letter of each phrase under the Section of the "P" in SOAP where it belongs.

Phrases

A. Perform an electrocardiogram (EKG).
B. Sample rectal contents via swab for parvovirus ELISA test.
C. Initiate loading dose of phenobarbital.
D. Prescribe phenoxybenzamine.
E. Place an IV catheter in the right cephalic vein.
F. Collect urine via cystocentesis.
G. Submit blood cultures.
H. Administer IV fluid therapy at maintenance rate.
I. Medicate with sucralfate tablets, 1/4 tab crushed in a slurry of water.
J. Review ear cytology.
K. Inject 2 units of glargine insulin SQ BID.
L. Order a urinalysis.

Section of the "P" in SOAP

1. Diagnostic plan . . . .
2. Therapeutic plan . . . .

Exercise 21: Considering Diagnostic Recommendations Further

The following phrases are typical of those that may be included in the "Diagnostic Recommendations" section of the "P" in SOAP.

Each phrase is missing one or more key details.

Identify what content is missing.

1. Repeat serum biochemistry panel . . . .
    . . . .

2. Perform ACTH stim test. . . . .
    . . . .

3. Perform thoracic radiographs . . . .
    . . . .

4. Perform a dexamethasone suppression test . . . .
    . . . .

5. Perform abdominal imaging . . . .
    . . . .

Exercise 22: Considering Diagnostic Recommendations Further

The following phrases are typical of those that may be included in the "Diagnostic Recommendations" section of the "P" in SOAP.

Each phrase is missing one or more key details.

Identify what content is missing.

1. Submit urine for full urinalysis . . . .
    . . . .

2. Biopsy the cutaneous lesion . . . .
    . . . .

3. Recheck calcium levels. . . . .
    . . . .

4. Test for Lyme disease. . . . .
    . . . .

5. Measure blood pressure . . . .
    . . . .

Exercise 23: Considering Therapeutic Recommendations Further

The following phrases are typical of those that may be included in the "Therapeutic Recommendations" section of the "P" in SOAP.

Each phrase is missing one or more key details.

Identify what content is missing.

1. Place IV catheter . . . .

2. Reduce dietary intake . . . .

3. Place urinary catheter . . . .

4. Reduce body weight by 10% . . . .

5. Initiate physical therapy on day 1 post-op . . . .

Exercise 24: Considering Therapeutic Recommendations Further

The following phrases are typical of those that may be included in the "Therapeutic Recommendations" section of the "P" in SOAP.

Each phrase is missing one or more key details.

Identify what content is missing.

1. Administer IV fluid therapy . . . .

2. Submerse in lukewarm-to-cool, but not ice cold, water bath to lower core body temperature . . . .

3. Start the dietary supplement, glucosamine-chondroitin . . . .

4. Admit to the hospital . . . .

5. Administer liquid diet through feeding tube every six hours . . . .

Exercise 25: Creating a Problem List from the History

"Ginny," a 6-year-old intact female Bassett Hound presented for evaluation of a three-day history of vaginal discharge. The following are your notes from history-taking. Your task is to organize the key findings from these notes into a problem list:

Notes from History:

Owned since 12 weeks of age. Accidentally bred at 1 year of age, no resultant litter. Never re-bred. Typically in heat every six to seven months. Last cycle was six weeks ago. Noticed increased licking under tail a few days ago, then intermittent spotting on carpet after patient sat. Discharge is rust-brown in color to strawberry-pink. Foul odor. Increasing amount. Appetite has been "off" for the past week: less excited about eating? Doesn't finish meals. Vomited once – undigested food – last night. Drinking more? Can't seem to settle. Took temperature last night: 104.2°F. History of testing (+) *Anaplasma* on annual 4DX ELISA four months ago. Never symptomatic and not treated.

   Note that there may be more blank spaces than will be filled

   Note that in real-life cases, the problem list would not be completed until after performing the physical examination. In this exercise, we are intentionally creating the problem list prematurely, for the purpose of highlighting key points

Problem List:

   1. . . . .

   2. . . . .

   3. . . . .

   4. . . . .

   5. . . . .

   6. . . . .

   7. . . . .

   8. . . . .

   9. . . . .

   10. . . . .

Exercise 26: Creating a Problem List from the History

"Buster," a 3-year-old castrated male Border Collie presented for evaluation of a one-week history of intermittent head-shaking and pawing at the right ear. The following are your notes from history-taking. Your task is to organize the key findings from these notes into a problem list:

Notes from History:

Adopted six months ago from rescue organization. No prior medical history other than UTD on rabies and DA2PP vaccinations. Multi-pet household: two other dogs and one cat. No problems with integrating into household. Head-shaking first noticed by owner a week ago. Owner didn't think anything of it initially, but it hasn't gone away. May be getting worse. Now pawing at right ear. Occasionally cries when pawing at ear. Both ears look "gunky" but inside of right ear looks red to owner and warm to touch. No change in appetite or thirst. Increased dandruff noticed along topline. Scratches coat a lot "all over." Seems more "itchy" than other pets in household. Went swimming in pool 1.5 weeks ago. No history of at-home ear care.

    Note that there may be more blank spaces than will be filled*

    Note that in real-life cases, the problem list would not be completed until after performing the physical examination. In this exercise, we are intentionally creating the problem list prematurely, for the purpose of highlighting key points

Problem List:

1. . . . .

2. . . . .

3. . . . .

4. . . . .

5. . . . .

6. . . . .

7. . . . .

8. . . . .

9. . . . .

10. . . . .

Exercise 27: Looking at the Whole Picture: Where Does Information Belong?

The following phrases or statements are typical pieces of information that might appear in a SOAP note. For each phrase or sentence, write S, O, A, or P to indicate in which section of the SOAP note it belongs.

. . . . . .   1. Audibly congested with stertorous breathing.

. . . . . .   2. Indoor-only.

. . . . . .   3. Owner reports one-week history of sneezing.

. . . . . .   4. Upper respiratory infection.

. . . . . .   5. Began to open-mouth breathe halfway through examination.

. . . . . .   6. Reduced interest in eating kibble last night.

. . . . . .   7. Littermate is asymptomatic.

. . . . . .   8. Reportedly FeLV/FIV neg/neg per adoption records.

. . . . . .   9. Conjunctivitis OU.

. . . . . .   10. Owner says photophobia started today.

. . . . . .   11. Green-yellow, opaque, ropy nasal discharge sneezed onto exam room table.

. . . . . .   12. Marked conjunctivitis OU with epiphora.

. . . . . .   13. Administer saline nasal drops to both nostrils q 4 hrs PRN.

. . . . . .   14. Ocular discharge began three days ago OD; it has since "spread" to OS.

. . . . . .   15. Pot-bellied, doughy abdomen with diffusely thickened, ropy loops of bowel.

. . . . . .   16. Moisten dry kibble with chicken broth or warm water to pique interest in eating.

. . . . . .   17. Ate warmed canned kitten food this morning.

. . . . . .   18. Start oral antibiotics [brand _____] at a dose of _____mL PO BID.

. . . . . .   19. Adult feline housemate started sneezing yesterday.

. . . . . .   20. Flea dirt at tail base.

Exercise 28: Looking at the Whole Picture: Where Does Information Belong?

The following phrases or statements are typical pieces of information that might appear in a SOAP note. For each phrase or sentence, write S, O, A, or P to indicate in which section of the SOAP note it belongs.

...... 1. On examination, patient has a right-sided head tilt.

...... 2. Owner says patient is disoriented.

...... 3. No known access to rodenticides.

...... 4. Owner noticed circling behavior at home this morning.

...... 5. Nystagmus with fast-phase to right.

...... 6. R/O central vestibular syndrome.

...... 7. No CP deficits as long as weight is supported.

...... 8. Submit CBC/Chem/UA.

...... 9. Owner not sure if patient sustained trauma overnight.

...... 10. Patient did not eat breakfast.

...... 11. Otoscopic examination AU WNL.

...... 12. Consult with anesthesiologist regarding anesthetic protocol.

...... 13. R/O CNS space-occupying lesion.

...... 14. Patient is kenneled outdoors overnight.

...... 15. Perform MRI of the CNS.

...... 16. Changed brand of commercial dog food two days ago.

...... 17. Ptyalism.

...... 18. R/O meningitis.

...... 19. Patient was groomed last week via a mobile clinic.

...... 20. Patient vomited this morning.

Exercise 29: Creating a Clinical SOAP from Scratch

Consider the following scenario:

A 2-year-old female spayed Great Dane presents on emergency after ingesting one-half to three-quarters of a bag of mixed milk and dark chocolates. The chocolates were individually wrapped in foil. When the client got home from work 45 minutes ago, he inadvertently left the chocolates on the counter. The ingestion happened when he stepped out of the room to change out of work clothes. The client attempted to induce emesis with a 1/4 cup of hydrogen peroxide. The dog did not vomit. On presentation, the dog is bright, alert, and responsive. The dog's breath smells like chocolate. Physical examination is unremarkable except for the following incidental findings: mild tartar at the upper canines, elbow calluses, and an engorged tick at the dorsal aspect of the leading margin of the right pinna. Given the history of ingestion, you prophylactically induce emesis by crushing a 6 mg tablet of apomorphine, mixing it with sterile saline, and squirting it into the conjunctival sac. Within five minutes, the dog vomits a large amount of kibble and chocolate, much of which is still covered in foil. You flush the conjunctival sac and provide the owner with the option to either admit the patient for overnight observation and IV fluids (dilution is the solution to pollution) or discharge home with supportive care (bland diet tonight and tomorrow; famotidine 10 mg PO BID). The client elects the latter and agrees to return if over the next 24 hours, the dog develops hyperactivity, persistent vomiting, diarrhea, or muscle tremors. In the absence of these clinical signs, no recheck is indicated. You remind the client to keep all chocolate out of reach because chocolate toxicosis, particularly when involving dark chocolate or cocoa, can adversely impact not only the gastrointestinal tract, but also the heart and nervous system. You inquire if the patient receives any flea/tick preventative. The client answers in the negative. You convince him to start a monthly topical flea/tick preventative, which he purchases on his way out the door. You also ask that he monitor the elbow calluses for cracking or signs of irritation; unless these develop, no treatment is indicated.

Construct a clinical SOAP note from the material provided. For the purpose of this exercise, you do not need to provide differential diagnoses for each problem that you list in the "A" section of the SOAP note.

S:
O:
A:
P:

Exercise 30: Creating a Clinical SOAP from Scratch

Consider the following scenario:

A 3-month-old intact female Russian Blue cat presents to you to establish a veterinary–client–patient relationship, one week after being purchased from an out-of-state (TX) cattery. The patient was driven by car to current home state (AZ), where client is a student in the college of veterinary medicine. The client intends to take the kitten on road trips to Seattle, WA, and also by plane to upstate NY on university-scheduled breaks. The kitten is indoor-only and is the only pet in the household. There are no plans to expand the household's pet population. The kitten eats commercial kitten chow. She is fed as much as she will eat. Her intake is not measured. She uses the litter box without issue. She has produced formed stool. Vaccination records were left at home. History of being dewormed, but product name, date of administration, and amount of product given were on vaccination records. Owner to scan in and send via email later this afternoon. Client elects to hold off on any vaccinations until records have been reviewed. On physical examination, she is bright, alert, and responsive with a body condition score of 3/9. She has a 2 × 5 mm region of periocular hypotrichosis dorsal to OD as well as a 2 × 3 mm alopecic patch on the dorsal aspect of the right carpus. There are crusts along the perimeter of the carpal lesion. She has a 5 mm reducible umbilical hernia. She has age-appropriate mixed dentition, and a pot-bellied appearance to her abdomen, which palpates as doughy, with thickened, ropy loops of small intestine. The remainder of her examination is unremarkable. You discuss with the client your suspicions about ringworm, and recommend that you perform a Wood's lamp examination and pluck fur for a fungal culture. You discuss the umbilical hernia and the client elects to monitor over time for it enlarging, becoming non-reducible, or becoming painful to the touch. If the umbilical hernia is still present at the time of ovariohysterectomy, the owner agrees with your recommendation for surgical correction. You recommend that a fecal sample be submitted for analysis and you discuss kitten-specific care, including nutrition. You recommend microchipping, flea/tick/ heartworm preventative, and that the client start at-home dental care and nail trimmings.

Construct a clinical SOAP note from the material provided. For the purpose of this exercise, you do not need to provide differential diagnoses for each problem that you list in the "A" section of the SOAP note.

S:
O:
A:
P:

Answer Key for Exercises

Exercise 1: History-Taking

1. C   6. C
2. O   7. O
3. O   8. O
4. C   9. C
5. C   10. C

Exercise 2: Transforming Closed-Ended Questions into Open-Ended Questions or Statements

1. Describe Edward's energy level.
2. Tell me everything that you feed Edward, beginning with the first thing he ate for breakfast yesterday morning and ending with the last thing he ate before bedtime.
3. Describe your flea/tick prevention plan for Edward.
4. Tell me about Edward's vaccination history.
5. Share with me what you do to maintain Edward's hygiene.
6. Share with me how it was that Peeta came into your life.
7. Tell me about Peeta's urine.
8. Please describe Peeta's attempts to urinate.
9. Tell me about Peeta's appetite.
10. Tell me about Peeta's lifestyle concerning his exposure to other cats.

Exercise 3: A Detailed Approach to History-Taking

1. Which brand of food?
    How much do you feed at each meal?
    Other than meals, what else does she eat every day?

2. Which brand of flea/tick preventative?
    How often do you give flea/tick preventative?
    Do you administer flea/tick preventative seasonally or year-round?
    What is the route of administration (i.e. oral, topical, . . .)

3. Which vaccines has Tulip received?
    When were these vaccines administered?
    When do these vaccines expire?
    How were these vaccines administered (i.e. subcutaneous route of administration vs. oral vs. intranasal)?

4. Where did Christopher come from?
    Did you adopt Christopher from a shelter or a private home?
    What is Christopher's vaccine history?
    Were you given a copy of Christopher's medical record?

5. What brand of litter?
    Is the litter scented?
    Is your cat using the litter box?

Exercise 4: Breaking Down the "S" in SOAP

1. B, I, O
2. K, N
3. E, J

4. Q
5. C, G
6. F, P, R

7. A, M
8. D, H, L

Exercise 5: Breaking Down the "S" in SOAP

1. J, M, Q
2. A, G, L
3. D, K

4. F
5. H
6. B, E, P

7. I, R
8. C, N, O

Exercise 6: Breaking Down the "S" in SOAP

1. D, G, N, R
2. B, J, P
3. E, L
4. H, Q

5. A
6. C, I, K, O
7. F
8. M

Exercise 7: Breaking Down the "S" in SOAP

1. D, I, O
2. E, K, M, Q
3. C, F, R
4. N/A

5. B
6. A, P
7. G, J, N
8. H, L

Exercise 8: "S" vs. "O"

1. Objective
2. Subjective
3. Subjective
4. Objective
5. Objective

6. Subjective
7. Subjective
8. Objective
9. Subjective or Objective
10. Subjective

Exercise 9: "S" vs. "O"

1. Subjective
2. Subjective
3. Objective
4. Subjective or Objective
5. Objective

6. Subjective
7. Subjective or Objective
8. Objective
9. Objective
10. Subjective

Exercise 10: "S" vs. "O"

1. Subjective
2. Objective
3. Subjective
4. Objective
5. Subjective

6. Subjective
7. Objective
8. Subjective
9. Subjective
10. Objective

Exercise 11: "S" vs. "O"

1. Subjective
2. Objective
3. Subjective
4. Objective
5. Objective

6. Subjective
7. Objective
8. Objective
9. Subjective
10. Subjective

Exercise 12: "S" vs. "O"

1. C
2. B
3. E
4. B
5. A

Exercise 13: Conversion Factors for Body Weight as Listed in the "O" Section of SOAP Notes – Part 1

1. 5.6 kg
2. 2.3 kg
3. 11.4 kg
4. 0.9 kg
5. 3.6 kg

6. 34.1 kg
7. 56.8 kg
8. 70.9 kg
9. 37.3 kg
10. 29.1 kg

Exercise 14: Conversion Factors for Body Weight as Listed in the "O" Section of SOAP Notes – Part 2

1. 28.6 lb
2. 41.8 lb
3. 50.6 lb
4. 114.4 lb
5. 11 lb

6. 63.8 lb
7. 140.8 lb
8. 24.2 lb
9. 4.4 lb
10. 83.6 lb

Exercise 15: Conversion Factors for Body Weight as Listed in the "O" Section of SOAP Notes – Part 3

1. Higher
2. Higher
3. Lower
4. Higher
5. Higher

6. Lower
7. Lower
8. Lower
9. Higher
10. Lower

Exercise 16: Breaking Down the "A" in SOAP

1. A, C, L
2. D, J, M
3. E, G, H
4. B, E, F, I
5. H, K

Exercise 17: Breaking Down the "A" in SOAP

1. D, H, L
2. B, C, E, K

3. G, I, J
4. A, E, F, M

Exercise 18: Breaking Down the "A" in SOAP

1. D, F, J, M
2. B, E
3. A, C, H, L
4. G, I, K

Exercise 19: Breaking Down the "P" in SOAP

1. A, C, D, F, G, H, J
2. B, E, I, K, L

Exercise 20: Breaking Down the "P" in SOAP

3. A, B, F, G, J, L
4. C, D, E, H, I, K

Exercise 21: Considering Diagnostic Recommendations Further

1. *When* is the test to be repeated? Six hours from now? Two days from now? A week from now?
2. *What* is the test's protocol? *Which* injectable agent is being used: ACTH gel IM or Cortrosyn IV?
3. *Which* radiographs? A lateral view only? A D/V view? V/D? Two-view? Three-view?
4. *What* is the test's protocol? Is this a low-dose suppression test or a high-dose suppression test?
5. *Which* kind of imaging? Radiography? Ultrasonography?

Exercise 22: Considering Diagnostic Recommendations Further

1. *Which* urine? Free catch urine? Sterile urine, as collected by cystocentesis?
2. *Which* lesion? *Where* is the location of the lesion? Specific details about the lesion would be helpful. Also: *how to biopsy?* Is an excisional biopsy expected? Or incisional? Punch biopsy? Wedge biopsy?
3. *Which* calcium levels? The calcium that is measured in a serum biochemistry panel? Or ionized calcium?
4. *Which* test for Lyme disease? A 4DX ELISA snap test? Lyme Quant C6 test? Lyme Multiplex test?
5. *Which* blood pressure? Mean arterial pressure? Systolic blood pressure? Diastolic blood pressure? Also: *using which technique?* Doppler or oscillometric?

Exercise 23: Considering Therapeutic Recommendations Further

1. *Where* is catheter to be placed? Right cephalic vein? Left lateral saphenous vein? Also: *what size* catheter?
2. *How* is intake going to be reduced? *By what amount?* i.e. Reduce each meal from 2 cups to 1.75 cups, for a total of two meals and a total of 3.5 cups per day.
3. *What type* of urinary catheter? *Which size?*
4. *What is the goal? By when* should body weight be reduced? One month from now? Two months from now? A year from now? Also: *how* will body weight be monitored? At-home? In-clinic?
5. *What type* of physical therapy? Range of motion exercises? Gait training? Aquatic therapy?

Exercise 24: Considering Therapeutic Recommendations Further

1. *What type* of IV fluid? *At what rate?* Any fluid additives?
2. *What* are we cooling the body to? *At which temperature* do we discontinue cooling?
3. *What* is the correct dose for the patient? *Is there a specific brand* that you are recommending? What is the appropriate dosing frequency?
4. *What* is the anticipated stay in the hospital? Overnight monitoring? Three to five days? Also: *where* within the facility? Intensive care? Isolation ward?
5. *How much?* Milliliters? Kcal? Also: *which brand?*

Exercise 25: Creating a Problem List from the History

1. Intact female
2. In estrus six weeks ago
3. Progressive vulvar discharge × 3 days: malodorous, rust-brown/strawberry-pink
4. Febrile
5. Off-appetite
6. Increased thirst
7. Vomiting – 1x
8. Restless
9. History of exposure to *Anaplasma* – (+) ELISA snap test

Exercise 26: Creating a Problem List from the History

1. Head-shaking × 1 week
2. Pawing at right ear (AD)
3. Painful AD?
4. Red AD?
5. Aural discharge AU?
6. Excessive dandruff – topline?
7. Pruritus?
8. History of swimming 1.5 weeks ago

The question marks acknowledge that these are problems based upon what the owner has described. These findings have not yet been confirmed on physical examination.

Exercise 27: Looking at the Whole Picture: Where Does Information Belong?

1. O	5. O	9. A or O	13. P	17. S
2. S	6. S	10. S	14. S	18. P
3. S	7. S	11. O	15. A or O	19. S
4. A	8. S	12. A or O	16. P	20. O

Exercise 28: Looking at the Whole Picture: Where Does Information Belong?

1. O	5. A or O	9. S	13. A	17. A or O
2. S	6. A	10. S	14. S	18. A
3. S	7. O	11. O	15. P	19. S
4. S	8. P	12. P	16. S	20. S

Exercise 29: Creating a Clinical SOAP from Scratch

S:

2 yr FS Great Dane

CC: chocolate ingestion ~45 min ago: milk and dark, individually foil-wrapped, approx. 1/2 – 3/4 bag

O attempted V+ with 1/4c H_2O_2 PO – unsuccessful at inducing emesis
Not currently on flea/tick preventative

O:

GA: BAR
INTEG: Bilateral elbow calluses; engorged tick – dorsal aspect of leading margin AD
E/E/N/T: NSF
CV/RESP: NSF
GI: Mild calculus – R and L maxillary canines; chocolate smell to breath
URO: WNL
LN: NSF
MS: NSF
NEURO: WNL

A:

Problem List:

1. Chocolate ingestion
2. Engorged tick AD
3. Bilateral elbow calluses

Diagnostic Plan:

1. Apomorphine (6mg) – 1 tablet crushed, mixed with sterile saline, squirted into conjunctival sac; successfully induced V+ of kibble, chocolate, foil

Therapeutic Plan:

1. See apomorphine notes above. Conjunctival sac then flushed
2. Bland diet, tonight and tomorrow
3. Famotidine (10 mg) – 1 T PO BID, beginning tonight
4. Start monthly flea/tick preventative
5. Monitor calluses for cracking or irritation; otherwise no treatment indicated

Client Communication Notes:

1. Reviewed the dangers assoc. with chocolate toxicosis including adverse impacts on GI, CV, and NEURO systems. Can cause V/D, tachycardia, arrhythmias, muscle hyperexcitability, tics, tremors, and potentially seizures. The darker the chocolate, the greater the danger
2. Options include:

   - Plan A: admit for overnight observation and IV fluid therapy to dilute any of the active ingredients that were observed
   - Plan B: discharge home to the care of the client; client to monitor; will return on emergency if over the next 24 hrs, the dog develops hyperactivity, persistent vomiting, diarrhea, or muscle tremors.

3. Owner opts for Plan B
4. Remind owner to keep all chocolate out of reach
5. Reviewed potential for tick-borne disease. Patient should receive monthly flea/tick preventatives. O elects to start monthly topical product. Purchased 12mo. supply

Exercise 30: Creating a Clinical SOAP from Scratch

S:

3 mo FI Russian Blue kitten
CC: new patient visit

PPHx: Purchased 1wk ago from TX cattery; drove by car here to AZ (where currently resides), plans to travel by car to Seattle, WA, and via plane to upstate NY

No other pets at home
Eats commercial kitten kibble ad libitum
Normal litter box habits; O has witnessed formed stool
Vx records and deworming history at home; O says will email records today

O:

GA: BAR, BCS 3/9
INTEG:

1. 2 × 5 mm region of periocular hypotrichosis dorsal to OD
2. 2 × 3 mm alopecic patch on dorsal aspect of R carpus with crusting along perimeter
3. 5 mm reducible umbilical hernia

E/E/N/T: NSF
CV/RESP: NSF
GI: age-appropriate mixed dentition; pot-bellied appearance to her abdomen, which palpates as doughy, with thickened, ropy loops of small intestine
URO: WNL
LN: NSF
MS: NSF
NEURO: WNL

A:

Problem List:

1. Periocular hypotrichosis – dorsal to OD
2. Alopecic patch with crusting – dorsal R carpus
3. Reducible umbilical hernia
4. Doughy, pot-bellied abdomen
5. Diffusely thickened ropes of small bowel
6. Underweight
7. Unknown FeLV/FIV status
8. Unknown vaccination history
9. Unknown deworming status

Diagnostic Plan:

1. Wood's lamp to evaluate for dermatophytosis
2. Fungal culture to confirm dermatophytosis (a negative Wood's lamp does not R/O dermatophyte)
3. FeLV/FIV ELISA snap test to establish serological status

Therapeutic Plan:

1. Calculate caloric intake for RER based upon ideal body weight
2. Monitor umbilical hernia at every visit

Client Communication Notes:

1. Owner to scan in and email vx records and deworming history by the end of work-day today. Still advised client to submit fecal sample for analysis.
2. Will discuss vaccination recommendations with owner once previous medical records have been received and reviewed
3. Recommend OVH once patient has received core vaccinations
4. Owner to monitor umbilical hernia for increased size, becoming non-reducible, and/or becoming painful. Sx repair will be performed if still present at time of OVH
5. Discussed benefits of microchipping with owner
6. Discussed benefits of flea/tick and heartworm preventative
7. Discussed at-home dental care – start brushing teeth now
8. Discussed at-home nail care – start trimming now

Appendix 3

Additional Resources That Provide Guidance for Record-Keeping

U.S. Resources

Accredited Veterinary Colleges
https://www.avma.org/ProfessionalDevelopment/Education/Accreditation/Colleges/Pages/colleges-accredited.aspx

American Association of Veterinary State Boards
https://www.aavsb.org/
https://www.aavsb.org/OurServices/look-up-a-license

American Veterinary Medical Association (AVMA)
https://www.avma.org/Pages/home.aspx

AVMA Model Veterinary Practice Act
https://www.avma.org/KB/Policies/Pages/Model-Veterinary-Practice-Act.aspx?PF=1

Medical Retention Laws by State
https://www.avma.org/Advocacy/StateAndLocal/Pages/sr-records-retention.aspx

State Summaries Regarding Confidentiality of Medical Records
https://www.avma.org/Advocacy/StateAndLocal/Pages/sr-confidentiality-patient-records.aspx

State Veterinary Medical Associations
https://www.avma.org/advocacy/stateandlocal/statevma/pages/default.aspx

U.K. Resources

British Small Animal Veterinary Association
https://www.bsava.com/

Clinical and Client Records
https://www.rcvs.org.uk/advice-and-guidance/code-of-professional-conduct-for-veterinary-surgeons/supporting-guidance/clinical-and-client-records/

Code of Professional Conduct for Veterinary Surgeons and Supporting Guidance
https://www.rcvs.org.uk/advice-and-guidance/code-of-professional-conduct-for-veterinary-surgeons/pdf/

Keeping Veterinary Medicine Records
https://www.businesscompanion.info/en/quick-guides/animals-and-agriculture/keeping-veterinary-medicine-records

Record Keeping and Audits
https://www.bsava.com/Resources/Veterinary-resources/Medicines-Guide/Record-keeping-and-audits

Record Keeping for Veterinary Medicinal Products
http://adlib.everysite.co.uk/resources/000/264/395/VMGNote16.pdf

Record Keeping Requirements for Veterinary Medicine
https://www.gov.uk/guidance/record-keeping-requirements-for-veterinary-medicines

Canadian Resources

British Columbia Veterinary Medical Association
https://cvbc.ca/Files/Bylaws-Policies/Bylaws_App_A_-_Code_of_Ethics_Oct_091.pdf

Canadian Veterinary Medical Association
https://www.canadianveterinarians.net/policy-advocacy/documenting-abuse-cases

Guide to the Professional Practice Standard
https://cvo.org/CVO/media/College-of-Veterinarians-of-Ontario/Resources%20and%20Publications/Professional%20Practice%20Standards/MRGuide2015.pdf

Index